Th 30/30 Body Blueprint

How Just 30 Minutes For 30 Days
Sets You Up For Unlimited Energy,
Easy Weight Loss and an Inspiring Life

Tim Drummond & Phil Hawksworth

RETHINK PRESS

The 30/30 Body Blueprint
Published in Great Britain 2013
by Rethink Press (www.rethinkpress.com)

© Copyright Tim Drummond & Phil Hawksworth
Front cover design by www.basecreative.co.uk

Contents

Introduction

It's 5.30am.
Your alarm clock is blaring next to you and you need to drag yourself out of bed again.
After hitting snooze a few times, you're eventually up, dressed, showered and ready to go by 7am.
Glancing in the fridge as you whirlwind through the kitchen… there is no food in, so breakfast on the move again.
No delays – perfect.
You have 10 minutes to nip in to the café for a croissant before getting to the office.
And a coffee, of course.
A big one.

By mid-morning you feel ravenous and head over to the vending machine for a sugar fix.
10 minutes and a heavy burden of guilt later, you regret eating the sweets… a fruit smoothie will balance it out.
Work is crazy.
This is five weeks straight of 10 to12 hour days and you are certainly feeling the stress.
By 12.30pm you're on your third large coffee: you feel wired and jittery but still like you could close your eyes and relax, and be asleep in the time it took you to face-plant the desk.

Lunch with colleagues is on the cards.
Still feeling guilty from the sweets earlier, a sandwich seems a good option, nice and healthy.
Wash that down with some Diet Coke, no calories so that's ok.
By the end of it you're feeling great, you didn't succumb to anything unhealthy and your friends witnessed your will power too.
Bonus!

Around mid-afternoon you are really flagging.
Knowing it's going to be another late evening, you take some down time and browse the internet.

Looking for answers as to why you feel lethargic and struggle to concentrate around this time every day.

By 7pm you are finished up at the office and decide to head down to the gym. Sweaty, overcrowded and generally an uncomfortable place for you to be. Pitch a tent on the end treadmill for an hour.
Just get the time in, trudging along slowly whilst craning up at the drivel on the TVs.

By the time you arrive home it is 9.30pm.
Tired, hungry and all in all a bit grumpy.
You drag a microwave meal out of the freezer and collapse on the sofa.
At least you can take solace in knowing that you did your hour of cardio.
That's three times already this week.

After some TV, texting and internetting, you head off to bed and lie staring at the ceiling.
Not being able to sleep is the most frustrating thing.
You know you're tired, you are being worked to the bone, but you cannot switch off.
Glancing at the clock, the alarm is set for six hours' time...
five and a half hours' time...
five hours...

Does this sound something like your typical day? If you can pick pieces out of this little story and identify some that sound like your life, this book is going to help you.

What to expect

Research from NASA says that habits take 30 days to create.
That's why the first period of this life-changing plan is a single month.
Just 30 days.

This is all we want you to concentrate on for now.
You will have some work at the beginning, looking at the long-term aims.
That is always the starting point.
Then that will be put on the backburner and we dive in for the first 30 days.

Ask yourself now, can you focus for the next 30 days? Can you make some changes to your health and fitness, move your nutrition and training up your list of priorities, and start to offer evidence that you can do this? Find a long-term answer to the constant ups and downs of dieting, fitness gimmicks and frustration.

It is proven that actions can become habits in 30 days.
Achieve for that initial period and the rest will come so much more easily.

Expect to feel amazing by the end of the 30 days, both mentally and physically.
Sure, you will drop that dress size which may be up there with your aims and goals, but it will be way more than that.
Our process is a simple, step-by step-guide, which will transform your health, mind and body.
When you reach the end of the 30 days, we challenge you not to be proud of the change you feel, inside and out.

How the 30/30 Body Blueprint works

The 30/30 Body Blueprint is both based in scientific research and, most importantly, works in the real world.

Here is what hundreds of hours of research showed us:

Screw willpower... Habits rule!

Willpower does not work in losing weight.
Diets do not work either.
People using their willpower to try and diet are still overweight, obese, unhealthy and now unhappy to boot!

Habits rule because they work with the way our brains are built, not against it.
We have the most complex piece of computing power on earth in our heads.
Yet not one of the major diets out there has ever seemed to study how this works.

Willpower is reliant on the conscious brain.
Habits on the subconscious brain.
In the long term, the subconscious is the boss.

What if we were to say that if you did something which takes 30 minutes for the next 30 days, the likelihood of you reaching your long term health and fitness goals would increase by 50%...
Would you be up for that?

Sure you would.

This is what we found when researching books and studies of mindset and success: If you do something every day for 30 days it becomes engrained as a habit.
Don't just believe us, believe NASA.
They are the super brains who found this to be true.
We just took their research, applied it to real world problems and gave it to you to create the answer to your health and weight struggles.

NASA found that after 30 days of repeating an action, new neural pathways were created.
A habit became embedded.
We became 'unconsciously competent' – which means we can do something without thinking about the process as we do it. As children we learn the process of climbing stairs until we are unconsciously competent at it. Now that action becomes harder if we try to think about the process we go through to climb stairs.

In other words, our brains actually change.
Our thoughts and therefore our behaviours change with it.
When achieving this, we go from willpower and conscious struggle and effort…
To unconscious habit, confidence and ease.
You become unconsciously competent!

Do what we suggest for those 30 days.
Not only have you increased the likelihood that this will stick…
You will feel amazing.

Your skin will shine.
Your energy levels will go through the roof.
You will feel your confidence go sky high.
You will be stronger and fitter.
And that dress size you've been trying to lose will drop off before your very eyes.

And that will all stick.
Permanently, in unconscious competency.

Ask yourself how many times you have tried this before…
Has it ever stuck?
Maybe not.
30 minutes for 30 days is all that we ask.
Be smarter and this is the last time you will ever have to try to achieve your goals!

Problems with the Women's Fitness Industry

- The Tracy Anderson paradox – people are extremely busy these days. Between a career, family, an active social life and household chores it seems there is no free time to fit in working out or thinking about the other factors influencing your health and fitness. Not a good place to be, considering experts tell you to 'work out six days a week for 90 minutes at a time'.

- Instant gratificationitis – our technological society has made people extremely impatient. We are used to everything being delivered instantly, this second, and expect to treat our bodies in the same way. Unfortunately there is no magic pill for better health and a better body.

- The airbrush – the media and advertising are always drilling into your head an image of 'what you should look like' and trying to sell you products based on this short term, surface appearance, often to the detriment of your health and even your medium to long term appearance. Sex and vanity sell and there are plenty of people out there willing to take advantage of that.

- Lies, lies, lies – You're told that if you buy this (insert crappy exercise equipment or shake diet) you will wake up the next morning with the body of your dreams. To compound this, the 'experts' and government agencies often give you advice that is out-dated and disproven. This accumulates to create confusion, misunderstanding and overwhelm, and makes it hard to know where to start on this journey.

- 'Get a Jessica Ennis body in six weeks' – celebrities and athletes are often held up as the standard in magazine headlines and replicating what they do will make you look as healthy, fit and vibrant as them. Of course this just requires working out for three hours daily, having a personal chef and daily afternoon naps. Clearly, this is not an actionable plan even if it was going to work for you. There is a lack of realistic, attainable and achievable plans out there that will take you to where you want to be.

- The 'detox' problem – people bounce between periods of being highly motivated and being 100% strict on everything, and the complete opposite, bingeing and almost purposely harming themselves. Having feelings of deprivation and wanting instant gratification is a recipe for disaster. Consistency and doing the right thing, the majority of the time, doesn't sit well with a lot of modern belief systems.

How this book will help

- Everything is based on 30 minutes a day, and is easily manageable to fit within your lifestyle and schedule. We give you the resources and knowledge to be able to plan and structure your life so that it is sustainable and becomes a normal routine. You brush your teeth every day, right? It's a habit. Preparing a healthy lunch for tomorrow can become a habit too.

- You will delve down deeper into your basic values and beliefs, and understand what it is that you really want, and why you want it. With this knowledge you set sensible goals that you can attain steadily and consistently before progressing to the next stage, your next goal.

- We encourage you to define what you wish to attain: how you want to look, how you want to act and how you want to feel. There is no preconceived ideal of how you should be. It is totally up to you and about taking you from where you are now, to where you want to be. Strong, fit, healthy, vibrant and energetic.

- We give you enough information for you to have a decent understanding of why you are doing what you are doing, why it works and, more importantly, to empower you to judge and make choices for yourself. You will understand what is right and what is wrong with your plan, and have the power to know how to respond to outside influences.

- Everything we suggest is attainable and achievable for almost anybody. There will be no outrageous hunger or constant exercising. Just small and simple steps that fit easily in your day, making it all very realistic and sustainable. Consistency is what will create change and ultimately bring about the results that you desire.

- Consistency comes from the mind, understanding and believing in what you are doing, why you are doing it, and what you will achieve by doing so. This is fundamental to our principles: you as an individual are empowered to set your own path. There is no expectation that you must 'do what we say'; rather we hope you will build up consistency by working on whatever you need to work on at the level you are at.

What to do with this book

"To know and not do, is to not know"

Stephen Covey

Use this book in a practical way.
As you read through the book you should scribble on it, do the exercises there and then, visit the resources online, make notes and schedule things in your planner.
Do it on the first read through, so as not to forget.

Pick it up on your commute, in the bath or for half an hour before bed, but do it every day.
Submerge yourself in it for a week to really allow all the information to sink in, whilst going through the exercises and creating changes in your life.

Within the first few pages you will find a practical exercise that will already start moving you in the right direction towards achieving your goals.

This book is written from our experience of working with thousands of women who have faced many of the same problems, beliefs and struggles as you may have, and have overcome them and achieved their desires.

If you commit now to undertaking all the exercises in this book, follow them and consistently practise the steps, you will achieve your health and fitness goals, whatever they are.
You will have a manageable and easy to follow plan that fits around your existing lifestyle, that is enjoyable for you to follow and that manifests the outcomes that you hope for, whether they are improved strength, confidence, sports performance, weight loss, illness management or much more.

The Five Pillars Model

The five pillars model is a representation of the five aspects that contribute to your health and fitness. We know they work because we use this model at Arete Fitness.

The pillar model indicates that each is of equal importance and the integrity of the whole is based upon the combination of all five parts working in synergy.

Weakness in one or more of the pillars will weaken the whole structure.

Pillar 1 – Mindset/Emotion
Pillar 2 – Nutrition
Pillar 3 – Lifestyle
Pillar 4 – Exercise
Pillar 5 – Habits

Mindset/Emotion

Mindset/Emotion represents the fundamental thinking and beliefs that you hold relating to yourself, your body, food, exercise, and many other things. Included within this area would be:

- Your values and beliefs

- Goals and progress measurement

- Perspective

- Motivations

- Responsibility

- Accountability

- Self-belief and confidence

- Perseverance

Nutrition

Nutrition is not 'a diet' but it is your long term eating patterns. How certain foods affect your body, what you should and should not eat and how to do so. Included within this area would be:

- A general definition of what constitutes good and bad quality food

- Breaking the 'dieting' model and focusing on your life-long eating plan — or why dieting does not work

- Understanding the reasons for focusing on food quality rather than quantity

- Learning the practical basics of nutritional biochemistry

- Food science

- What to eat

- What not to eat

- How to structure your eating

- Supplementation

Lifestyle

Lifestyle is everything physical that affects your health that is not diet or exercise. How these things impact you and what to do to improve them. Included within this area would be:

- Stress

- Sleep

- Recovery

- Fun and play

- Relaxation and mindfulness

- Products

Exercise

Exercise doesn't have to be painful, dull and invasive. Just 30 minutes, three times a week is enough to achieve great results when you train right. Included within this area would be:

- Consistently challenging yourself to progress

- Prioritising lifting weights and getting stronger

- Enjoying the process of working out and not obsessing on outcomes

- Looking after mobility and doing gentle exercise like yoga

- Making working out a fun and social experience

Habits

Everything above builds into this element.
Most of your thoughts, actions and reactions are subconscious habits that your brain takes care of without your conscious input. This is a very powerful function and you need to harness it to help you, rather than let it hinder you. Included within this area would be:

- Preparation

- Setting your daily process goals to create new positive habits

- Logging and collecting data to understand current habits

- Avoiding willpower by having a good plan in place

- Accumulating little wins

- Being consistent

30 x 30

Habits are easy to make but hard to break, so try replacing old habits with new healthy ones.

It's initially hard to go against your natural urge, so make sure you always line up alternatives.

Create good habits to alter bad ones.

If you're feeling deprived you'll never achieve anything.

By creating good habits, you're focusing on the positive of what you are doing.

When you have a plan you usually end up falling into a habit without realising it.

If you say "my plan is to go to the gym three times this week before work" and you do this for a month, it becomes a habit and you no longer need to think about it.

New habits create new neural pathways and connections in your mind.

Habits are shortcuts so that you don't have to think; create a new pathway and it becomes subconscious and, once created, it's there and no longer a conscious decision.

You have taken it away from willpower.

Away from saying, "I know I should do… but I really want to…."

To achieve long term and sustainable results, you must create habits.

The habits must be achievable, rewarding and enjoyable.

When you follow our method, and use just 30 minutes per day, for 30 days, you create lifelong habits.

This will be the last time you need to get in bikini shape for summer, the last time you once again achieve a complete 10k run without stopping.

30 Minutes

You can almost always find 30 minutes in a day.

You probably spend that much time on Facebook…

When used appropriately, 30 minutes is plenty to achieve stellar results.

30 Days

Follow the plan for 30 days and you will have created a habit.

When it is a habit, it is easy.

You are now 'one of those people'.

Congratulations.

Case Study: Lauren

Lauren was stuck in something of a rut.

After a very active childhood, being involved in sports at a high level and loving life, the nine-to-five world was now starting to take its toll.

Of course, being London it was more like eight-to-eight most days, and now, in her mid-20s, she had lost some of her zest for life.

She gained a few kilos, her energy levels dropped and the pressures of corporate work in combination with a busy social life were all getting too much.

Lauren wanted to do something about it. She wanted to change and become 'her old self' again, but did not know where to start.

Not knowing quite what she wanted to achieve and not even nearly knowing how to get started or where to fit it all in led to… doing nothing.

Procrastinating and putting it off until 'it was less busy'. Like it was ever going to be less busy…

With a little bit of help understanding what it was that she wanted, and how to set some goals, Lauren started training with us at Arete.

She found that whilst she was extremely busy, she was able to set aside 30 minutes in the mornings before work, three times per week, to work out, and another 30 minutes on a weekend to prepare food and get ready for the week.

Her personality type made the training sessions perfect for her; as a very social person her motivation came from interacting with those around her. She wanted to understand nutrition and lifestyle on a deeper level , so she read the materials we provided, and worked with them to optimise her hormonal balance.

Balancing hormones – predominantly through avoiding sugar and grains to control insulin – led to her energy increasing once more, sleep quality improving and an easy road to dropping those few kilos.

But this wasn't the end.

Lauren had achieved her original goals; she had dropped some weight and upped her energy levels once more. Now she was into it.

Now she was the type of person who loves working out and she began working towards a number of strength and performance-based goals.

This was now something she thoroughly enjoyed – a part of her lifestyle.

Lauren is currently working on completing her first pull up – An impressive feat of strength for any woman to achieve.

You can see how Lauren has covered all five pillars: setting goals at the start, working on hormonal balance through nutrition and lifestyle, exercising socially, whilst getting stronger, and preparing and getting in to a habit to ensure consistency.

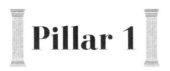

Pillar 1

Get your head right

Your brain rules your body.
And yet people insist on trying to change their health or appearance
(read: body) without even thinking about their mind (brain)!
Silly, right?
Silly indeed.

Case Study: Diane

Diane is in her mid-40s and working in a top management job at an investment bank.
Married with a teenage child, she had been focused on climbing the career ladder, and her health and fitness since having her child had deteriorated.

With an important job and a child to take care of, Diane was about as busy as it got.
She has client lunches a couple of times a week, is often in the office until gone 9pm and has an hour commute home.
She has access to almost every excuse possible for why she is not managing her health and fitness.

Indeed for many years she used these excuses to justify to herself why she wasn't doing anything about it.

Then came a realisation, on the back of a succession of illnesses that really took it out of her, that she needed to get back in to shape.
Her health was seriously suffering and she could not go on like this.
The stresses of life were causing anxiety attacks and she just did not feel young any more.

This was one of those 'life changing realisations' that comes about on its own.

The point at which you realise, this is it, I am going to make a change and nothing is going to stop me.

She knew she was going to do something about it, so Diane took action immediately.
She joined the gym near her office the next day and hired a personal trainer.
She knew that without this accountability she would likely not be able to commit to getting out of the office and down to the gym.

With the help and knowledge of her trainer, Diane educated herself about her eating choices and committed fully to making a change.
The turn-around was dramatic and in no time at all weight was falling off, she felt better, had more energy and stopped getting ill so often.
This all came from a commitment.
She was ready at this stage of her life, and she created the accountability that ensured she stayed on track with her goals.

Sometimes she would waver from what she was supposed to be doing – Diane is human after all! But keeping a food diary and tracking her compliance, then comparing that to her changing measurements allowed her to see when she was straying, and to work out how much leeway she had before it started negatively affecting her.

Exercise, it turned out, became something of a stress relief and she was glad to get out of the office a couple of times a week.
She never dreamed of looking like a fitness model, she just wanted to feel fitter and healthier again, and to be back to the shape she was pre-childbirth.

She now maintains the healthy eating, stress management and exercise as her normal.
She feels so much better; why would she not?

The first pillar of the Arete Fitness process is Mindset/Emotions, and there is good reason for this.

Without addressing the needs and wants, values, beliefs and ideas in your mind it doesn't matter what you do in terms of diet and exercise.
You're not coming from the right place and either will not do the right things, or you will start, but won't sustain them.
Why?

Because you don't know what you want, or why you are doing it.
Of course you will tell yourself that you do, everyone does.
But what you tell yourself is typically not relevant nor truthful.
Taking an objective view of their own behaviours is one of the hardest things for human beings to do.

You must understand your beliefs and values, determine your goals and limitations, and only then think about the implementation.
You need this foundation and knowledge to build upon when devising a plan to follow.

THE BIGGEST MINDSET MISTAKES THAT YOU MAY HAVE MADE IN THE PAST

- Not understanding your deep values and beliefs

- Having a short term, surface-level motivation

- Not setting goals

- Not taking responsibility for outcomes

- Not creating accountability

- Giving up when it gets hard

- Lacking self confidence

---

30 SECOND TAKE-AWAY TIPS

- You must understand your values and align your goals with them; this is what drives you, deep down.

- Motivation wanes – 90% of people who join the gym never achieve their goals. You need to have a purpose based on your values and the goals that you have set.

- Your 'plan' is determined from your goals, not the other way around. Figure out what your goals are and then work backwards on what you need to do to achieve that.

- You are 100% responsible for you. Excuses are worthless; if you cannot change something then simply accept it as a limitation and move on with what you can control. Do not beat yourself up about stuff that is not in your control. Work on the things that you can change.

- Change is hard; you must persevere and view failure as a lesson. As the adage goes perseverance is the key to achieving anything that is worth achieving. Hard work gets great results.

- Be accountable to yourself and others. Tell people what you are doing, keep records and measure progress.

- Believe in yourself!

Ok, we are going to jump straight in.

Values

Your health and fitness is essentially a reflection of your values.
Healthy people care about their health.
Crazy, *non*?

Your underlying values rule your actions, and whatever you do is based, on a subconscious level, on what your values are.
Your values embody your self-image, or self-identity.

Make a lifestyle choice

Most of your life takes place on a subconscious level.
This can be good… or bad.
It is basically impossible to fight your values, certainly not for a sustained period of time.

You always revert back to your fundamental beliefs and values.
You do things subconsciously, like you always have done.

So change needs to be a lifestyle choice.
Health needs to be a lifestyle choice.
Fitness needs to be a lifestyle choice.
Heck, looking good naked needs to be a lifestyle choice.
It just doesn't work as a flitting interest.
Or Januaryitis*

*Januaryitis – the phenomenon of transitory fitness obsession infecting the masses each January.

Positive > Negative

Every single thing you do is either moving you forwards or backwards; toward your goals, or away from them.
There is nothing in between.
Think about that…
So, if it is not positive, it is by definition negative.
Balance and moderation is destructive. Everything is cumulative.
If you want to achieve things, you have to be taking positive actions the majority of the time to bring the results that you want.
The positive must outweigh the negative.

So what is important to you?

Don't skip over it…
What is important to you?

Few people ask this question of themselves.
Fewer still really delve down into the answer.
Successful people do.
You can see in the case study that Diane did.

Do This: My Life Story (page 133)

- Set aside half an hour.

- Find somewhere quiet where you can relax and think in comfort, without interruption.

- Grab a pen and paper (real old-fashioned paper, not your tablet).

- Write your life story, from the perspective of yourself aged 60.

- Just start writing, and keep going until you have nothing else to say. This mental exercise is a very powerful tool for learning about yourself and your values.

- Don't think too much, or try to be too logical. Just let the emotion flow and guide the pen across the page.

SUGGESTIONS TO WRITE ABOUT:

- What is life like?
- What have you achieved?
- What are you proud of?
- What do you regret?
- What makes you happy?
- What makes you sad?
- How is your health?
- What are your hobbies?
- What one thing would you tell yourself in retrospect?

- Read back on your life story and see what jumps out at you.

- Does anything surprise you?

- How do you feel about this person?

You should be more aware of your wants and values after doing this exercise.
You can watch a video explanation and read an example story for this exercise on www.aretefitness.co.uk/lifestory
If it is important you are more likely to enjoy it.
When you value your health and care about how you feel, it won't feel like such a chore.
You will be motivated to do it simply because you want to take good care of yourself.
Doing what you want to be doing will naturally be enjoyable.
It will become part of your life.
Not something you force yourself to do because you don't enjoy it. You'll be doing something you genuinely want to do for a long time.
It won't be a fleeting interest or a passing hobby.
It will become an intrinsic part of your routine.
When you enjoy it, you are doing it for the right reasons.
You're going to find it a lot easier…
It becomes default.

Heaven forbid there might be a group of people who:
Love looking after themselves
Love working out
Love making and eating good food
Love setting and achieving goals
Love overcoming challenges
Love and are fully confident in themselves
Love helping others live a healthier life
Love socialising with a group of like-minded people

Purpose

'I want to get fit' is not enough.
Do you want to get fit so you can feel stronger and more confident?
But why do you want to feel stronger and more confident? Getting fit in itself isn't of value, but it's a means to a value.
To feel good about yourself.
To be comfortable with yourself.
This is your purpose.
Whatever you intend to do needs to fit with your values.

Once you're doing something in line with your values, you will have long term motivation.

It becomes your *purpose*.

You will enjoy it much more and be more motivated if you're going through a series of steps which will lead to your ultimate fulfilment and the life that you want to lead.

You are working towards something beautiful.

To be successful, your health needs to be viewed as equally important to the other things that you hold dear , such as your family and your career.

Some people are so driven by their need for hedonic instant gratification that they just want to get drunk and eat pizza every day, to the detriment of their health and career.

They 'want to have fun'.

When this person goes through a stage of deciding to get fit, they will likely not enjoy it, nor stick with it for very long.

Unless of course their outlook on life changes.

Goals first, plan second

Ever started a new exercise regime or diet plan on a spur of the moment decision?

Ever started anything on a spur of the moment decision?

How did it go?

Probably not well…

Goals

For it to go well next time, you need a more structured approach.

It's great that you started.

That is often the hardest step.

However, you also need to know where you are going!

Then you can work out how you will get there.

Define your goals first, then work out a plan based on the goals.

You will need something tangible to measure, to ensure you are making progress.

Make it congruent

Many decide to get fit or lose weight, but don't think about the whole picture, they don't consider how it fits in with their values or with their current lifestyle.
It leads to failure.
Have you been here before?
It's very easy to just think, 'Let's start' without thinking about what you're doing, or why, or what you're trying to achieve.
Nor how it fits in with your life.
Easy, however, is not always best.
You need to know why you want it before you can begin re-organising your life.
It's a chore and not very exciting, maybe even a bit boring…
But it leads to you *actually achieving* what you want.
That is what you want, right?
Take a step back and assess before getting too carried away.

Realistic and meaningful

You often see someone who is highly motivated and overexcited.
They have a short attention span, jump in head first, and it goes great.
It's January, they are armed with their resolutions and enough will power to do a juice fast for a week.
Magic.
Until…
A week or two later they get fed up and move on to the next big thing.
Failure, in double quick time.
The next wacky diet craze or something different all together.
'Forgetting' they ever even wanted to get fit.
If they'd sat down and thought about *why* they wanted it, and their core values on a deeper level, they'd be much more likely to succeed.
They could then determine some realistic and meaningful goals.
This is a platform to work from, to create a sustainable solution.

Decide why you're doing what you're doing before you decide how.
Set your goals, then work backwards to figure out the best course of action.

Once you know your 'why', then you can define your 'what' and then you can define your 'how'.
Why?
What?
How?

Why?

Articulate why you want to do something.
What gets you out of bed every day?
Knowing your 'why?' underpins actually doing it.
Your 'why?' is the instructions that are going on subconsciously.

What?

Tangible.
Measureable.
Meaningful.

How?

Create a plan.
Write down where you are now and where you want to be in the future.
Write down what has stopped you before and what you perceive could stop you this time.
Just thinking about it and committing it to paper is often enough to overcome a lot of these obstacles.

Do This: The Bridge Model

- Where are you now?

- Where do you want to be?

- What are your obstacles?

The 5 Pillar Method

Where you are now?　　　　　　Where you want to be?

What's stopping you?

Do This: Write your long term goals (Page 138)

- You just established them in the 'where do you want to be now'

- Write them down with the prefix 'I will…'

- Keep these somewhere that you will see them regularly: your bedroom, desk or stick them to your fridge or wardrobe. You want to have them in your mind on a regular basis.

Do This: Define what you are going to measure (Page 138)

- Based on your goals, what do you need to measure to track your progress?

- Measure it now as your starting point.

- Re-measure every two to four weeks

Process Goals

Set short term goals based on what your long term goals are.
You've made your plan for the long term outcome.
Short term goals should be based on the implementation of the plan.
'I will…'
Achievement of the defined processes will create the outcome that you want, if you have been implementing it properly.
If it doesn't, you know your plan is not right for you and you need to change it.

Small wins

Reward achievement of the process goals.
Small wins.

All about the small wins.
Process goal: Go to the gym at least twice weekly for the next four weeks.
Reward: Book a massage.
You have an incentive for the short term.
It breaks it down in to manageable pieces.
If your long term goal is a long way off it can seem insurmountable and you can lose interest.
Breaking it down keeps you progressing forwards
One step at a time.

Measure stuff

You need to know what you're trying to achieve so that you can measure it.
Measuring allows you to track your progress.
To know if you're going in the right direction.
So work out your goal and make sure you track your progress!

Tweak for you

There are many more similarities than differences in the way the body works so the big picture stuff will be the same for everyone.
That is just right or wrong, black or white.

However your situation and life is unique.
This is the thing that needs to be accounted for.
It will affect what you plan to do.
What is realistic, feasible and doable?
What is enjoyable?

Version 2.0

Not making the progress you want?
Modify your plan.
This only works if you followed a plan in the first place.
If you don't measure anything, if you don't even really know what you want, how do you actually know if you're making progress or not?
Once you've got something to measure, you can then look at the efficacy of the plan.

It takes away the grey area.
This is working for me. This is not working for me.

Responsibility

On a scale of 1-10 how important is this to you?
Is it more important than eating pizza?
Is it more important to you than getting pissed three times a week?
It doesn't have to be a 10 (out of 10).
It might be a 10 for a while, but in the moment you lose sight of what is realistic in the long run.
Commit to a manageable aim.
If your career is more important to you than health and fitness, that is absolutely fine.
Fit it in around your work, in a manageable way.
Understand how your fitness can add to your career.
More energy and concentration.
Setting goals, persevering, learning and achieving.
By admitting this now it is no longer an excuse.
It empowers you to take action to do something about it.
Now you have a realistic expectation and knowledge of a potential barrier.
Now your goals and plan will reflect this.

Do This: Commitment sheet Part 1 (Page 143)

- Take your 'I will…' statements from the previous exercise and expand upon them by adding in a completion date.

- Now write 'To achieve this goal I will…' and put in the process goals you must meet, these might be daily or weekly goals that are within your control. Do not write outcome goals at this point.

- You will add more to this sheet later on, keep it safe and in your mind ready for later.

You are 100% responsible for yourself.

People who blame genetics or having big bones or a busy schedule are in denial.

They are making excuses for their failure to take decisive action.

Of course those things count, and they are important:

Yes your schedule is busy – no denying that.

That is a fact and it is not going to change…

So work around it!

You are working to *be the best that you can be*.

Take responsibility and make a change that fits with your schedule.

It sounds obvious, stupidly so, yet people refuse to do it.

Time and time again.

They actively look for an excuse for why they are not going to be able to achieve something.

What kind of mindset is that?

Look for the way that you *will* achieve it!

We don't want to be too harsh on people who are suffering from this self-sabotaging.

Of course, they don't actually want to do it to themselves.

They just do not know any different.

Sometimes it takes a harsh word to make you face up to reality.

Change is hard

Change will bring results.

Change your action and the outcome will change.

As Einstein put it, '**Insanity: Doing the same thing, over and over again, and expecting a different result.**'

People have excuses and blame everyone else and everything else, but you determine your own actions.

Only you.

It's often not easy.

But it is in your control.

Making excuses or blaming others won't help you.

It might make you feel better in the short term but will make you feel worse in the long term.

To genuinely embrace change, you need to be on the edge of your comfort zone.

It's not easy.
That is what you must do to achieve your dreams.

Lessons

You only fail when you give up.
Setbacks are lessons.
Anybody who ever achieved anything of note had setbacks along the way.
It is the perseverance through hardship that separates the best from the failures.
Look to people who have come back from great tragedy, overcome great adversity and come out on top in the end.
Think of Nelson Mandela, Tanni Grey-Thompson, Steven Hawking.
Those who give up when the going gets tough are not the achievers.

Accountability

Create personal and social accountability by telling people what you are up to.
It is essential to keep you on track.
Without accountability, you will make excuses, life will get in the way and you will eventually fail.
Sounds harsh?
Life can be harsh…
Change is hard.
The results are worth it.

Mark Twain – **'Twenty years from now you will be more disappointed by the things you didn't do, rather than the things that you did.'**
You need to tell people what you are doing (social accountability).
Define what you are planning to achieve and put it out there in the public sphere.
One way to do this is visit www.aretefitness.co.uk/goalboard
This creates an expectation from them; they are waiting for you to manifest the changes you have spoken of.
It keeps it in your mind.
They will ask how you are getting on and encourage you along the way.
Nobody likes to go against their word.
You are subconsciously manipulating yourself (in a good way).

Watch out for saboteurs

One caveat: people close to you may try to rubbish what you are doing.
Tell you that you can't do it, or that you shouldn't be doing it.
Ignore them.
They are not being malicious.
Just projecting their own insecurities onto you.
It makes them feel bad when the people around them are picking themselves up and achieving things, whilst they're stuck in the same place.
Make sure you don't entertain their negativity and that you avoid talking about it with any people like this.
There are plenty of people about who will build you up, encourage you and help you.
These are the people you should be accountable to.
Find people who thrive in the area you are looking to address.
They will encourage you.

Do This: Commitment Sheet Part 2 (Page 143)

- Take your commitment sheet that you filled in earlier.

- Sign each process goal, and then have somebody else co-sign it.

- This is creating accountability to somebody else. Make sure it is someone who is important in your life, somebody whose opinion you value and who you will see on a regular basis.

- Even if they forget all about it and never say another word about it, subconsciously you will be accountable to them, and not want to disappoint them.

Do This: Blog about it

- This one is optional, but a great idea that we highly encourage.

- If you really want to keep yourself accountable, blog about your journey.

- Create a blog, do it on your existing blog, or microblog on Twitter or Tumblr.

- This is a great way to learn about yourself, motivate yourself, remain accountable and receive support and motivation.

- You will find that as other people read about your journey you inspire them. This is the most positively reinforcing motivation you will ever receive.

Self-Belief

Your attitude and belief is much more important than having the perfect plan.
Planning is important, but of course your belief and your attitude is the key.
No plan will be successful without it.
It's common and normal to want the perfect, super-duper plan straight away that will turn anybody into an Olympian in six weeks flat.
Problem is, even if that were possible (it's not), you would never follow it and maintain it.
Imagine the lengths you would have to go to.
You need something that is easy to follow.
Then you need to follow it.
It must be realistic for you and your life.
That is what we are all about, we help women to achieve the results they want in a way that is quick, easy and simple.
It is manageable.
It is possible.
For you and for anybody.
It is a lifestyle.

It is *female potential amplified.*
Henry Ford – '**Whether you think you can, or you think you cannot, you are right.**'
You are capable of whatever you think you are capable of.
If you believe in yourself, you can potentially achieve it.
It's not guaranteed, but if you don't believe in yourself it is guaranteed that you will fail.

Winning

How audacious your goals are dictates the likelihood of whether you will achieve them or not.
You might never be able to win a gold medal at the Olympics, but if you want it that badly and you dedicate your life to it, you're 98% there.
You cannot do anything more.
The rest is up to fate.
Regardless, your journey was infinitely more impressive than those who never started. Never tried.
Failing like this isn't a bad thing.
Failing like this is beautiful.
It means you tried something so crazy, with the odds stacked against you, but it just was not possible.
You are still unfathomably better than when you started.
That is more important.
That is what counts.
That is winning.

Whatever you dedicate yourself to, you have a fighting chance of achieving.
What you tell yourself and reinforce in your mind will come to fruition.
If you say you can't do it, it's too hard, I'm not good enough, guess what?
It's true!

Believe

Self-belief in conjunction with your values rules your actions.
When people don't believe they can do something, they won't.
They will mess it up to prove to the world, or themselves, that they can't do it.

Not on a conscious level – at least not usually – but subconsciously this is what is happening.

You can literally talk yourself into failure.

With the best will, the best facilities, the best plan and all of your other ducks in a row just waiting for you to succeed.

Keep telling yourself you cannot do it, and you will manage to f@#k it up.

Change is hard

People are keen to do something when it's easy.

They tend to stop doing something as soon as it gets hard.

We all want a magic pill!

We are hard-wired to prioritise short term gain over long term gain.

You must be prepared to make sacrifices.

Change is hard and it is painful, but it is necessary for achievement.

The hardest thing about change is disrupting habits.

Focus for a short period (30 days) on creating new habits and you have created change permanently.

Something has to give. There has to be a sacrifice on one side of the fence.

You cannot live a contradictory, incongruent lifestyle.

Either quit eating pizza and getting drunk every night, or give up your goals of having a flat stomach.

They just do not go hand in hand.

If you're not getting instant gratification from it, which you likely won't, especially in terms of your health, it's very easy to give up.

The reward for being healthy is the absence of ill health, so there's not necessarily even a visible or quantifiable reward. This is why it must be a value choice.

You *want* to be healthy.

For no reason other than that you care about your health.

Perseverance

Persevering is key.

No one ever achieved anything great when it's easy going.

The hard stuff counts.

Keep doing something, keep moving forwards.

You need to modify the plan if it's not working, but don't give up on it.

Modify and make minor adjustments until you find the formula that does work.

When times are tough, winners are made; there will always be a hump or a point where it gets hard.
Once you are over the hump, it will become easier.
You will have beaten it.
You know what? The satisfaction of achievement makes it more than worthwhile.

CHECKLIST

Have you:
- ✓ **Written your Life Story**
- ✓ **Completed the Bridge Model**
- ✓ **Re-written your Long Term Goals**
- ✓ **Completed the two parts of the Commitment Sheet**
- ✓ **Started blogging about your Journey**

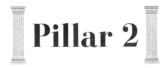

Pillar 2

Eat Real Food

Diet and nutrition can be an overwhelming and confusing subject.
There are a huge number of people out there giving often contradictory advice.
It can be difficult for the average person to make any sense of it all.
We feel that everyone should have some basic education in this field to be empowered to make informed decisions for themselves.
It is a fundamental aspect of looking after yourself and your family.
The responsibility is currently on the individual to find out for themselves.
We feel that more should be done to educate everyone.
However, as it is, you are responsible for you.

Case Study: Tracy

Tracy is a great example of someone who was in the right mind-set from day one.

She had made the decision that she needed to drop the weight she was holding after having her child and was ready and willing to do what was necessary.

All that she needed now was to learn a framework that allowed her to make the right choices when it came to her eating habits.

Some education about what to eat and what not to eat, and how to structure that in to meals and she was on her way.

Tracy dived in head first and made quite a big change to her normal eating habits whilst she was highly motivated.

During this time, whilst simultaneously training at the gym and getting stronger and toned, she consistently lost a couple of pounds each week.

Once she was at her goal weight she was able to maintain healthy eating patterns, because she realised that there was more to it than just weight.

Health is important to her and for this reason she has struck a nice balance of eating great, nutritious food as her baseline.

When she is going out, or when she fancies it, she can deviate from this a bit.

This allows her to enjoy what she is doing and not have it consume her.

Of course, if she indulges for a couple of weeks – like when on holiday – she quickly spots things beginning to go in the wrong direction and a couple of weeks tightening things up soon puts an end to it.

She generally has ham and berries for breakfast, varied salads for lunch and a lot of home cooked dishes for dinner, along with snacking on nuts.

Nothing too fancy, just simple and quick food that works with her lifestyle.

THE BIGGEST NUTRITION MISTAKES THAT YOU MAY HAVE MADE (MOST ARE NOT YOUR FAULT!)

- Being influenced by advertising and not educating yourself about nutrition

- Following fad diets

- Eating too little and calorie restricting

- Eating a low fat diet and not enough protein

- Eating too much soya, grains and sugar

- Falling into the trap of junk foods that are labelled as health foods

30 SECOND TAKEAWAY TIPS

- Unprocessed food is real food and should always be the focus of your diet

- Get away from thinking of 'dieting'. Your diet is just the food that you eat, it needn't have any correlation with trying to lose weight. We refer to our nutrition guidelines as an 'eating plan' to try and break this association.

- Calories are just a unit of energy and counting them is redundant. Eating the right foods is all you need to worry about and the calories will take care of themselves.

- Learn what to eat and what to avoid, and then focus on what you are eating. Get away from the feeling of deprivation when you're not having certain foods and focus on all of the great stuff you can have.

- Food quality is the only really important factor. Find the best quality food you possibly can. This is your health we are talking about.

- Supplementing can be a great way to fill in some of the missing pieces you cannot get through your food intake. Do not be afraid to add in some high quality supplements to optimise your health.

- Food scientists manufacture food to be as tasty and addictive as possible to the detriment of your health. You receive little to no actual nutrition through these processed 'foods' so your body stays hungry, craving more nutrients.

Many people do what advertising tells them to do.
Not your fault, but not a good idea.
Certain popular diet clubs say you can eat anything as long as it doesn't contain a high number of calories, and millions of women subscribe to this notion.
Eat shit and (try) to stay a bit hungry.
That's healthy, right?
Many of us purchase low fat products because we believe they're better for us and will help us lose weight.
Low fat anything is actually much worse for you than the full fat version.
'Low fat' is a marketing ploy that people fall for.

The same goes for fake meat and soya products.

Just eat meat like human kind have for millions of years.

If you're a vegetarian for health reasons, replacing meat (real food) with processed crap is nonsensical.

Soya-based proteins are very disruptive for your body.

Despite claims to the contrary, wholegrains are not a health food.

Calling something 'whole' does not automatically make it good for you.

Grains just aren't great for you.

They are very likely to cause an inflammatory reaction in your stomach, causing bloating and puffiness.

For example, breakfast cereal is crammed full of wholegrains, sugar and low fat vegetable oils

It is not going to be good for you! Grains, sugar and vegetable oils make up the triumvirate of 'crap I should not eat'.

Vegetable oils and margarine made from plants and highly processed to be edible are, in fact, extremely unhealthy.

Natural fats from animals, coconut or olives are the ones that are good for you.

Diet drinks and smoothies: liquidised fruit takes away all the fibre and leaves sugary liquid.

Diet drinks removing sugar and adding in chemical crap.

No, no, no!

Fad diets.

Living off watermelons or cabbage soup.

No.

Surefire way to tank your metabolism and give yourself long term health concerns and guaranteed rebound weight.

You get fatter by doing this amazing weight loss diet…

Yet this is what you are told you need to do to lose weight.

This is what is pedalled to you.

It really is not your fault.

Your granny was right

Natural and unprocessed food is the key to good health.
One hundred years ago people generally had the right idea.
They ate good, honest, whole foods.
The processed food prevalent in modern western diets today did not exist when your grandmother was young.
Literally did not exist.
How can something that has only existed for a few years be healthy, be what the human body is designed to eat?
The concept is ridiculous.

No processing and manipulation of 'food'.
This wasn't a conscious health decision; it was simply all that was available.
These days, due to advances in science, when we think we're eating healthy 'food', a lot of the time we're not actually eating food at all...
Not really.
Food, by definition, must nourish the body.
Something containing just empty calories and nothing that enriches you (and probably stuff that has the opposite effect) is not really food.
'Food-like substances'.

The basic food groups which we recommend you should eat:

- Meat

- Fish

- Eggs

- Fruits

- Vegetables

- Dairy (in its natural state, non-pasteurised; we don't advocate milk)

- Animal fats: butter, lard, tallow, etc.

- Nuts

- Seeds

Do This: Read the 'Real Food Guidelines' (Page 134)

Macronutrients

Food is made up of different macronutrients: proteins, carbohydrates and fats.

Protein and fat are the essential macronutrients that you absolutely cannot live without.

You *can* live without carbohydrates.

That's not to say that you should, but they are not essential.

Protein and fat are crucial and humans cannot survive without them.

It's in vogue currently to follow a low carb diet, which is a fast way to lose weight.

If you are overweight it is a very simple way to get healthier.

However, if you are already lean it is probably not the best option for you.

Equally, if you have lost significant weight following a low carb diet it may be time to move to something more rounded.

At the end of the day it all comes down to food quality.

We will expand more on that later.

For now: If you want to lose weight, eat better quality, real foods and fewer carbohydrates.

Ketogenic diet

You may have heard that you can't survive without carbohydrates...

Not true.

If you eat no carbohydrates at all, your body shifts in to a state known as ketosis.

The misconception here is that without glucose coming in through eating carbohydrates, the body does not produce energy.

However ketone bodies are produced at an elevated level.

Ketone bodies are always present in the system and a lack of carbohydrates leads to an up-regulation of this system.
Your body shifts to a lipid-based metabolism when in ketosis.
Lipid = fat.
You start using fat as your primary energy source.
Sounds good…

Another point of confusion arises from the fact that the human brain requires glucose to function.
Which *is* true.
People often use this as a reason you must eat carbs.
Actually your brain can survive on ketone bodies and some glucose made through gluconeogenesis.
Gluconeogenesis is the production of glucose from proteins when the body is low on glucose.
The brain only requires about 20% of its energy from glucose.
This can easily be made from excess proteins.

Sugar

Sugar is the real enemy.
We just explained how your body is perfectly happy without it.
Sugar is what causes insulin resistance (diabetes).
Insulin resistance happens when your body over produces insulin, to ship sugar out of the blood stream, causing the receptors to desensitise and 'not listen', necessitating more insulin.

Leptin

Leptin is another hormone that obese people are shown to be resistant to.
Leptin is nicknamed the 'hunger hormone'.
The hunger hormone tells you when you are full.
Fructose; a component part of sugar is shown to inhibit leptin pathways.
Leptin resistance follows because whilst it is released, the body does not pick up the signal and therefore does not stop eating.
Hunger.

Carbs

There are different types of carbohydrates.
Glucose is a sugar, which is one molecule long.
Complex carbohydrates are multiple glucose molecules stuck together.
It all breaks down to become glucose in the body.
Complex carbs take longer to be broken down and absorbed.

Fibre is a type of carbohydrate.
Soluble and insoluble fibre.
Fibre is indigestible plant material; meaning it passes straight through your digestive system.

Soluble fibre dissolves in water and readily ferments in the gut, slowing the movement of food through the digestive system and thus the absorption rate.
This means it keeps you feeling full for longer.

Insoluble fibre does not dissolve in water, and acts as a bulking agent.
Helping to keep bowel movements regular and easy to pass.
Fundamental for a healthy gut; which is the key to the health of the whole body.
You need to be excreting waste.

Most vegetables and many fruits are mainly fibre, which is why there are basically no calories in them.
Then there are others that are mostly water, like cucumber or lettuce.
Cucumber has next to no energy in as it is 90+% water.
No matter what, it's vital to eat plenty of vegetables for a complete micronutrient profile and to get sufficient fibre.
Regardless of how low carb a diet you want to be on, you can still eat fibrous vegetables, especially green and colourful vegetables.
Opt for an array of different colours.
That adds a good variety of nutrients to your diet.

Stomach Health

The gut is key to the health of the whole body?
Indeed it is.

The gut lining is the biggest barrier between the outside world and the inside of your body.

It is where good stuff is absorbed and bad stuff is shut out.

80% of your immune system is in the gut.

The gut also produces many hormones and neurotransmitters.

For this reason it is sometimes called the 'second brain'.

If your gut is unhealthy, you are susceptible to many things.

Depression, for example, because the gut is home to serotonin: the 'happy hormone' (excuse the gross oversimplification).

Typical western logical medicine looks at depression as a psychological issue and never even considers a potential connection between the physiological body and the psyche.

Diet, exercise and lifestyle is often shown to be as, or more, effective than anti-depressants in research studies.

Auto-Immunity

Research recently is showing that a host of autoimmune diseases are caused by damage to the gut lining.

A predominant food that is implicated is gluten.

Gluten is a protein found in grains such as wheat, rye and barley.

Gluten is a very reactive protein that, it has been shown, damages the gut lining and is linked with not only autoimmunity, but also weight gain and mood disorders.

This is why we are strongly against eating gluten.

Some foods as a 'treat', such as sugar, are relatively benign when it's a one-time thing.

Gluten, however, even in small doses, can cause lasting problems.

A bit of icecream at dessert or a couple of squares of chocolate is cool as an occasional deal.

Donuts just are not.

Just don't eat that stuff.

You will be thankful.

Fats

Fat is a macronutrient group.

One with a very bad reputation.

It is unfortunate that the same word also means overweight.
It creates a lot of association and connotations that often are not justified.

Fat is essential for human life.
Your brain and nervous system are made up mostly of fat.
If you have too little fat in your diet, it can be deadly.

The same goes for cholesterol.
Very bad associations.
The fact is, cholesterol is what makes your cell membranes and sex hormones.
Sounds pretty essential doesn't it?
Yet everybody thinks it is bad!

Good Fat, Bad Fat

We don't like the term good and bad fat.
It's not that simple.
It's never that simple…
However, for simplicity we will reluctantly use the terms.

Our broad definition of a bad fat is one that's been processed.
Certain fats are very unstable.
Particularly vegetable fats, which are of course the ones being processed.
Unstable fats + processing = bad.

Saturated fats are more stable and typically come from animals.
Though there are exceptions.
Unsaturated fats are less stable and more susceptible to reactivity.

If you look at the molecular structure of lipids (fats), they have a carbon atom on the end.
Saturated fats have closed bonds, unsaturated fats have open carbon bonds.
Meaning they react very easily to air, light, heat, etc.
The more unsaturated a fat is, the more unstable it is because it has more open bonds.
Very boring, but…
This is why we recommend saturated fats for cooking.

Because they're very stable and don't denature easily.
Now you know.

Saturated fats

Saturated fats are typically animal fats and also coconut oil.
Coconut oil is kind of in a little world of its own.
Coconut oil is predominantly made up of medium change triglycerides (MCTs).
MCTs are absorbed through the gut much more easily than other fats.
They are very kind to the body and great for a variety of reasons.
So when cooking, use coconut or animal fats.
Butter, ghee, lard, tallow, duck fat, goose fat are all great and offer a variety of alternatives for different tastes and cuisines.

Why nothing can be wholly 'good' or 'bad'

Viewing the world in a very reductionist way where everything is either good or bad, black or white, is precisely the problem with Western 'health' industries.
This is why we prefer not to label things in such a way.
The fact is, everything is on a scale, somewhere towards one side or the other.
It is never binary.

Fats specifically…
Everything is a mixture of saturated, monounsaturated and polyunsaturated.
Nothing is only one or the other.
For example people who say butter is a saturated fat, are making a massive oversimplification.
Butter is *predominantly* saturated, but also has a massive chunk of monounsaturated fat.
The same stuff that makes olive oil 'so good'.

Monounsaturated fats

Monounsaturated basically means there's one open carbon bond; polyunsaturated means many open bonds.

Monounsaturated are more stable than poly, but not as stable as saturated fats.

Monounsaturated fats are proportionally high in foods like nuts and olives. This means they are ok for low temperature cooking such as baking or roasting.

Olive oil is a good example of that.

Olive oil is good to cook with at a low temperature or to eat cold, but it's not good to cook at very high temperatures with.

Don't fry your steaks in it.

Pour it on top of some roast veggies and stick them in the oven for 45 minutes, sure.

Dress your salad with it.

Polyunsaturated fats

Polyunsaturated fats are the most interesting.

They are essential for good health, but also potentially the most toxic.

There is definitely a lot of confusion about this and they are often labelled as 'healthy' across the board, which is just not the case.

As usual, it is more complex than that.

Polyunsaturated fats are the most volatile because they have many open bonds.

Oily fish are high in polyunsaturated fats and extremely healthy.

Possibly the ultimate health food.

Indeed, these fats are essential for good health and many people benefit hugely when they begin taking a fish oil supplement.

The two types of polyunsaturates that people predominantly talk about are Omega 3 and Omega 6.

There are literally thousands of research papers espousing benefits of these fats for any and every part of the body, illness or condition you can think of.

Omega 3s, if not denatured, are an essential part of the diet and very good for you.

Omega 6s are a little more tricky.

They are also essential.

However, people tend to overdose on them and have way too much in their diet.

This upsets the ratio of Omega 3 to 6.

It is the ratios that are important, rather than absolute amounts.
There are extremely high quantities of Omega 6 in grains, the meat of animals that are fed grains, and in vegetable oils.
These, unfortunately, make up the majority of the typical modern diet.
Full of processed food, wheat products and low quality meats.
This equals a heck of a lot (technical term) of Omega 6 in the average person's diet.

The reason supplementation of Omega 3 is so effective for so many people is not because more is better.
That is a common misconception in the health sphere.
It is because people are starting from a place with so much Omega 6, they are simply starting to redress the balance.
It has changed a couple of times, but the current recommendation is a ratio of 3:1 of Omega 6 : Omega 3.
Short term, high dose supplementation is going to be beneficial if you have had a bad diet and/or are overweight.
The two usually go together.
Someone who eats good, high quality real food for a sustained period will not need the supplementation.
You are taking out a massive chunk of Omega 6 from your diet so you have a good ratio naturally.
You don't want to go the other way with mega intake of Omega 3 and too little Omega 6.
This again shows why it is not as simple as 'good' and 'bad'.
Who are you and what is your situation?
What is good for you may not be good for someone else.

'Bad' fats

Processed vegetable oils are the one thing we can absolutely say *are* bad.
They are predominantly a type of polyunsaturated fat, which, as we mentioned previously, is extremely reactive at the best of times.
Products (and they are exactly that, not foods) made from corn, sunflower, cottonseed, sesame, canola and soybean oils are what we would define as vegetable oils.
Let the 80s health food mantras stop here.
We do not include olive and coconut oils as they are consumed in their natural forms (and are fruits, not vegetables).

The processing these oils go through from plant to supermarket shelf sounds unbelievable.

Bleached, heated, spun, and sieved.

It sounds like making plastic, right?

That is pretty much what is going on, in a chemical sense.

These 'foods' are almost the same make up chemically as plastics.

These 'foods' have no taste and no texture, no smell.

This is why they are perfect for putting in processed foods: they do their job binding or creating the correct 'mouth feel' without being detected with a smell or taste.

Find a processed food and it is pretty much guaranteed that one or more of these oils will be present.

Check the labels.

Not good.

They're also dirt cheap.

They originated as a by-product from other processes and were used in glamorous things such as paint and varnish.

When somebody realised they were 'edible', they could be marked up at a crazy percentage and sold.

Then we were brainwashed in to thinking they were actually good for us!

This is what a huge marketing budget and questionable ethics can achieve.

This is taking a worthless commodity and making it into a hugely profitable product at its finest.

Compared to natural fats, such as butter or coconut oil, they are still dirt cheap even with the mark-up.

Which is another reason why food manufacturers choose to use them in their products.

Protein, protein, protein

Protein should be the base of every meal.

Our suggestion: do not eat a meal without a protein source.

Protein is predominantly in meat, fish, eggs and dairy.

Other sources include beans, pulses and grains.

These would be secondary sources and shouldn't be relied on as a large part of your diet.

They're lower quality proteins, which have to be eaten in larger quantities to get the same amount of protein.
Stick with the meat, fish, eggs and dairy as your staples.

Protein is the most essential macronutrient to make a regular part of your diet.
The reason being, it is constantly turning over.
Cells die and regenerate all day, every day.
Protein is the building block for the whole body.
It's not just muscles, but bones, joints, hair, nails and everything else.
Look at most hair care products and they are full of amino acids (proteins).

Protein is the most 'filling' food.
You will be most satiated after eating a protein-based meal.
High quality sources are also some of the most tightly-packed sources of nutrients available.
Especially fat-soluble vitamins and trace minerals that are uncommon in plant foods.

We recommend protein is the first thing on your plate, and the rest of the meal is built around that.
Regardless of what your goals are.
It is fundamental.
Eat your protein.

Vegetarian diets

If you are following a vegetarian diet you need to ensure you meet your protein needs.
You need a full amino acid profile; you might have heard that you should mix rice with beans to meet your protein needs, for example.
Be careful that you do not fall in to the trap of thinking it is fine to eat anything (crap) as long as it is vegetarian.
Donuts on toast is a vegetarian meal…
It won't be good for you.

Tim: "I used to be a vegetarian. I was born into it and lived as a vegetarian for the first 20 years of my life. I realised, as I began researching more into nutrition that I was missing out on a lot and even potentially deficient in essential nutrients. Nowadays, I believe that it is a bad choice for your health to be vegetarian. Of course I can understand moral reasoning for doing it and that is very much up to the individual. What I do want to emphasise, though, is that you may be sacrificing your own health in doing so."

Some vegetarians are healthy and eat natural, healthy foods within the vegetarian paradigm.
That is great and, if it is what you choose to do, you should do ok with that.
But there is a misconception that by shunning meat you are instantly healthier.
Research that says vegetarians are healthier than the general population is flawed.
By being health conscious and taking a decision to address their eating habits they are so far ahead of the general population that of course they are likely to be healthier.
Although we would argue they have focused on the wrong factor in the study.
The general population is so unhealthy, it really is not saying much.
If they actually measured someone who ate meat and only natural foods, they would be healthier still.
But they don't.
That would be a *crazy* idea.
Vegetarians who live in sync with nature and only eat natural food and vegetables are generally in a much better place than most people, so go right ahead.

Dispelling the myths about saturated fat

People who sell food products containing saturated fats and animal products don't really have a marketing budget.
They're farmers.
A farmer who has a farm with a few cows and some sheep can't do much to persuade you to buy his product.
He is completely at the mercy of the supermarkets and middlemen distributors.
The multinational food corporations who manufacture vegetable oils and

processed foods have unfathomable amounts of money to spend on marketing, on guiding scientific research and on altering public and professional opinion.

Whose message gets out there...?

For a long time, the big food corporations have managed to direct the way science has been going.

The fact is, scientific research can only happen when someone pays for it.

These companies can, and do, do this.

There's no one on the opposite side to counteract.

The average farmer likely isn't going to fund a £500 million study.

But, hey, you never know…

Basically, they were directing the way that science went, which is why it was easy for them to convince everyone (including the government) and no one questioned it.

Remember the 'food pyramid'?

You were no doubt taught it in school.

This is what has been pushed to the public for years, on the back of questionable research.

Only recently, with the internet and the new flow and freedom of information, have the 'little people' had a voice.

Lots and lots of 'little people' with lots and lots of evidence have a growing voice, and public opinion is shifting.

For example…

Saturated fat isn't bad for you.

People ate saturated fat for a long time before scientists decided that we shouldn't eat it.

A natural animal product that human kind has eaten for millions of years.

Shunned for something that has been 'produced' in the last 50.

The logic here is astounding.

How can man think he can outsmart nature?

Evolution dictates what food is and what we need to survive and thrive.

Crazily enough, we evolved to eat animals, not paint (vegetable oils).

The China Study

In the 50s, scientists started looking for reasons why more people were getting fat, and investigating the dramatic increase in heart disease, diabetes and cancer.

A research paper came out called the China Study.

Its publisher, Ancel Benjamin Keys, was an American scientist who studied the influence of diet on health.

In particular, he hypothesised that different kinds of dietary fat had different effects on health.

His belief was that saturated fat was responsible for all of the world's dietary woes.

It was an 'easy fit'.

Eating fat makes you get fat, right?

It sounds logical. (It's not really if you understand how complex the human body is.)

Keys doctored the results and only showed half of the test subjects (countries) to make it fit his hypothesis.

This belief was embraced and went on to become the conventional wisdom.

Ever since, Keys has been something of a celebrity and the Western world's healthcare practitioners have been taught his hypothesis.

Doctors and dieticians have been taught that saturated fat is bad and that it makes you fat and sick, so instead we should eat 'healthy' vegetable oils. This is then fed down to their patients and through the media and official guidelines – the lovely food pyramid referred to above.

Food quality

Natural food is good and processed food is bad.

It's quite black and white; there are only a few caveats.

Carbs or fats are not bad; it's about the food quality.

Real food grows on trees and in the ground, or it runs and swims around.

Processed food is made in a factory and comes in plastic wrapping and sits on shelves for months on end without decomposing.

The fact is, your body needs food, real food.

The same as any animal needs food.

We're not different to, or somehow above, any other animals.

We just like to think that we are.
Our bodies need the same essential things:
Proteins, fats, fibre, water and an array of micronutrients.
They come as nature packaged them.
Humanity has eaten them for millions of years and as a species we've done just fine.

Man verses nature

In the last one hundred or so years, man has apparently outsmarted nature.
We have tried to make our own food.
Better and improved.
Food 2.0.
It is no coincidence that in this period obesity and lifestyle diseases have sky rocketed.
The stuff that you have no idea how it's made or even what is in it, is not real food.
If it's made in a factory in packaging with multiple tens of ingredients, then it's more than likely going to be processed and full of rubbish that's going to make you gain weight or become unwell.

Anything you could catch, find or make yourself is real food.
This will make you fit and healthy.

Soil quality

Unfortunately, even real foods nowadays are much less nutritious than they used to be.
It comes down predominantly to soil quality.
The land has been over-farmed and the soil itself has very little nutrition left.
Instead of nature being left to its own devices, or nomadic farming where farmers consistently move around, the same soil is used again and again.
Agriculture nowadays is all based in one spot, especially crop fields.
They just turn over the land so quickly, crops grow, take all the nutrition out, fertiliser is added back in to make up for the deficit.
Unfortunately, fertilising doesn't give a rounded nutrient profile – only enough to make the crop grow.

Survive, but not thrive.
Not to mention the environmental cost of using fossil fuels to achieve this 'fertilisation'.

In reality they shouldn't need fertiliser.
The ground should contain enough nutrients to handle vegetation.
Otherwise plants would not grow in that spot.
Because the soil is so depleted we have to use the fertiliser to grow things and we end up eating this nutrient-poor produce.
It's not just fruits and vegetables either; the animals that we eat are fed in this same way and it is an upward chain of poor nutrition.
The soil feeds the plants, which feed the animals, which feed us.
Or not, as the case is, because whilst we eat we are still hungry for nutrients.

Food displayability

The UK and US are the worst countries as consumers for being picky about food.
We want – or at least the supermarkets drive us to want – everything to be consistent.
Consistent size, shape, colour, flavour, and for the produce to not deteriorate quickly.
It is all about how it pleases our senses, rather than how it nourishes our bodies.
Just looking at the fruit and vegetables you can tell the difference.
You can see by the colour and the taste, when you visit other countries, that their fruit and vegetables are more nutritious.
In Britain, people expect vegetables to be a certain way and the 'odd' shaped ones don't get sold.
This is to our detriment; we have demanded that our own food becomes less healthy and nutritious.

Malnourishment

Recent research has shown that a lot of obese people are actually malnourished.
Yes, you read that right…
Experts have hypothesised that obesity is a state of malnourishment.

This is because obese people tend to eat processed food that contains so little nutritional value it's not really food and certainly is not nourishing their bodies.

They're eating lots of calories but they're not taking in any micronutrients or anything useful from it.

The body still needs more to be adequately nourished.

This is one of the reasons why obese people overeat.

There's no satiety signalling, so they never know when they're full.

The body just keeps crying out for more food, to nourish itself.

So they keep on eating.

Leptin resistance, playing out, as explained previously.

If you try and eat several plates of steak and broccoli you get full very quickly.

But you can sit and eat a packet of biscuits or a bag of crisps very easily and quickly.

Because they have no nutrition, but loads of calories, you don't receive any satiety signals and you can just keep gorging on it.

Not to mention that snack food is manufactured specifically to make you eat more and to be addictive.

It is hard to resist.

Food manufacturers add ingredients including sugar, salt, MSG and additives to make it more addictive, so you eat more and thus buy more.

You're over-caloried (again, probably not a real world), but under nourished.

Calories

A calorie is a unit of energy.

The definition of a calorie is: one calorie is the amount of energy needed to heat 100ml of water by one degree.

Most people don't know what a calorie is, they just know not to eat too many of them.

It's just a way of measuring energy, nothing more than that.

Therein lays its own limitation.

It doesn't tell you very much.

Calories are not all the same.

100 calories of donuts is not the same as 100 calories of eggs.

If you ate 1,000 calories of donuts a day you would gain weight.

If you ate 3,000 calories of eggs and broccoli a day, you would be pretty healthy and likely not gain weight.

It's not about how many calories you eat; it's about what they are and what you do with them.

Food quality, not quantity.

Note: We don't recommend living off just eggs and broccoli, either for nutrient balance or your sanity.

How your body really stores fat

100 calories of donuts is 100 calories your body will pretty much only store as fat.

It is worthless energy.

Broccoli, on the other hand, is full of fibre and nutrients, so 100 calories of broccoli will be absorbed in your body as useful energy and nutrition, which you put to use to build your body and burn off just simply by being alive and healthy.

It's not about the amount of calories, but where the calories come from that we need to consider.

Don't get confused…

If you eat 10,000 calories a day by just eating butter, you will gain weight and not be healthy.

We are talking about in a balanced, calorie appropriate diet.

Liquid calories

We also do not recommend liquid calories.

For example fruit juices and soft drinks.

It's very easy to drink 2,000 calories of apple juice and still be hungry and not even notice you've consumed anything.

You get lots of calories but, as you're not digesting it, it doesn't set off any satiety signalling.

Your body doesn't realise it has had food or energy and you still feel hungry.

Stick with water (lots of), coffee (not too much of) and teas (as you please).

The hunger games

Not being hungry is important.
When you're hungry you crave quick energy, and quick energy is usually junk food or liquids.
Then you get into that cycle of energy coming in with no nutrition, quickly getting hungry again and subsequently overeating.

Being hungry is not a good idea.
Restricting the amount of food you're eating is not a good idea.
That's not to say just eat everything with abandon.
Caloric consumption is relevant for certain things.
Unless you're an athlete, or someone already very lean looking for the last edge, if you are eating proper food, you just don't need to worry about calories.

Just eat good food until satiety.
When you're hungry again, eat again.
It can be liberating for those of you who have followed a number of different diets, counted calories and restricted yourself.

Just eat when you are hungry.
Until you are not hungry any more.
It is a beautiful place to be.
This is what it feels like to have a fully functioning leptin cycle.
Or, to put it another way, when you do not eat loads of sugar.

How to eat

Try and always sit down specifically to eat your meals.
Not at your desk or on the sofa.
If you've ever dined with a Japanese person, have you notice how they put their cutlery down between each mouthful?
It means they eat much more slowly and thus feel fuller from less food because leptin has time to do its job and tell your body that it has been fed.
Be mindful whilst eating.
Focus on the tastes and smells; focus on the act of chewing.
Try counting it out; they say you should chew foods up to 30 times.

Try it.

You will definitely slow down and become more aware of your eating habits.

Beyond being fat

It's not just about being overweight.

We hear a lot of people say, 'I'm not fat so I can get away with eating what I want.'

Unfortunately, it doesn't really work like that.

Just because you're not overweight, it doesn't mean you're healthy.

Being overweight is a sign of being unhealthy, but is not guaranteed.

Internally people can be falling apart, whilst externally not showing a lot of signs.

Unfortunately, we live in a hedonic society where a lot of people do not consider or care about their future health or anything but their current external appearance

Values.

We already covered it.

Eat the right foods, look after your lifestyle and exercise, and your risk of getting sick is considerably smaller.

Nobody wants to get ill.

Especially if it is potentially life-threatening.

Take action.

Look after yourself!

Of course, by eating crap whilst you are still thin, you are setting your body up to be extremely good at getting fat at some point in the future.

Know anybody who seemed to be slim for a long time, then reach a certain age and seemingly get exponentially bigger at an alarming rate?

Lifestyle diseases

Most common illnesses and diseases are partially lifestyle related.

Including cancer, heart disease, type 2 diabetes, many autoimmune diseases and the 'diseases of ageing', Parkinson's and Alzheimer's.

They now call Alzheimer's 'Type 3 diabetes', as it's related to too much sugar consumption and insulin dysfunction.

Because they're all lifestyle related, in theory they can be prevented, or at least the chance of contracting them greatly reduced.

You can drastically reduce your chances of getting these diseases by exercising regularly and eating healthy and nutritious food.

Most of these diseases rear their heads later in life and are typically far from the minds of young, 'healthy' people.

'Healthy' meaning not sick – as opposed to functioning optimally.

Although it might be far from your mind right now, if you value your health you should be thinking about the long term consequences of your diet and lifestyle.

Everyone thinks about their current situation, their today.

Smoking today doesn't quite compute to cancer in the future in our brains, even though we know full well that it is a distinct possibility.

What we do not consider is that our yesterday created our today.

By working in our today we can dictate what happens in our tomorrow.

You can take decisive action before the time.

Once you are fat and sick it is too late to change it.

You are fat and sick.

This is the power of the 30 days and creating a lifestyle habit.

You are creating consistency.

Family health

Pregnancy and breastfeeding is the most important time in a baby's life, healthwise.

What you eat and do while pregnant and breastfeeding is imperative for the baby's development and determines what they're going to be like for the rest of their life….

'The rest of their life'.

Genetic traits are turned on or off, it's called epigenetics.

Genetic traits with an environmental trigger.

This basically sets you up for life.

Obviously if you drink or do drugs when you're pregnant it's going to affect the baby.

Everybody knows that.

It is hardly difficult then, to understand that whatever else you are doing in your lifestyle will also affect the baby.

It's exactly the same if you eat unhealthy food.

The baby is eating what you are eating.
Whatever you do, you pass on to the baby.
A baby who has much smaller organs and a weaker immune system to deal with whatever is being thrown at it.
Anything that is bad for you is multiplied for a baby.
It is vital that you look after yourself in this period.

Organic?

Organic food is on the whole better for you, but it's not essential for following a healthy diet.
The term organic actually has mixed meanings, depending on what it is describing.
First we will address fruits and veggies.

Veggies

The definition of organic fruit or vegetables means the produce is not genetically modified and is grown without the use of pesticides or herbicides.
Pesticides and herbicides are toxins and should not be in the human diet. (Nor that of any of the other animals affected by this style of mass farming.)
Common sense indicates this is going to be healthier for you, avoiding those toxins.
It will typically be more nutrient dense also.
It's definitely worth opting for organic produce if you can afford it.
Farmers markets are a great place to source high quality produce that is much (much) cheaper than the supermarket.

Meats

Organic meat is a slightly different story.
In order to be considered organic, meat has to be reared without the use of hormones or unnecessary antibiotics and the animals have to be fed organic food.
No hormones and antibiotics is great, but…
This means the farmers can organically grow soy or wheat and feed it to the cows, and then the meat can be labelled organic.

The problem is, cows are not actually meant to eat anything much aside from grass.

The same thing that happens to us also happens to cows when they eat crap.

If a cow eats wheat, it gets fat and sick.

Its fatty acid ratios become distorted, which all means you're still not eating great quality meat.

For example, we mentioned the ratio of Omega 3:6 earlier.

To ensure your meat is optimum quality, opt for grass-fed or pasture-raised animals.

If you're shopping for beef or lamb, always look for grass-fed.

With pork, make sure it's pastured. With chicken, turkey or game, always opt for free-range birds, as well as eggs.

With most other animals, such as venison or less common meats, opt for wild.

Fish

When shopping for fish, you should look for fish that has been caught in the wild.

Farmed fish are the equivalent of farmed meats.

Fish farmers actually feed their fish wheat and soya.

Fish are clearly not supposed to eat wheat, as you'll never see a wheat plant in the sea!

Some fish farmers also feed their fish sawdust to bulk out the fish in the cheapest way possible.

Splendid.

Not, however, great for your health.

Generally, fish that are indigenous to Britain are not farmed as they're more prolific here, but if you can afford to buy wild fish, it's advisable.

You may pay a bit more, but by opting for wild you're not putting toxins and pesticides into your body.

Wild fish also taste a lot better!

Go to a farmers market or fishmonger to find reasonably priced wild fish.

Prioritise the most important things to spend the extra money on.

Vegetables that grow underground, such as onions or potatoes, are less exposed to pesticides and you needn't worry about them so much.

Fruits and above ground veg are much more heavily sprayed.

With meats, ensure that white meat like chicken is of better quality, especially if you are eating the skin.

If this is beyond your budget, do not worry about it.
Eating the right foods is still the most important thing and will take you most of the way.
The better quality of the same food is just optimising for that little bit extra.

Local support

If you shop at your local farmers markets, butchers, fishmongers and grocers, as well as being better for the environment and for your health, you will be supporting your local community and economy.
The profits go straight to the farmer instead of being eaten up by multiple middlemen and disproportionately shifted away from the ground level workers toward the suppliers and distributors (read supermarkets).
A reliance on fossil fuels to fertilise the ground sufficiently so things grow, combined with shipping foods in from the other side of the world because it is cheaper than sourcing them locally, is hardly good for the environment and will not be sustainable for too much longer.
Look closer to home for your meals.

The science of selling food

Food science is a massive industry in which food manufacturers use scientific methods to figure out how to make you eat more of whatever they're selling.
They work on texture and taste and smell and mouth feel and presentation to make you want to eat more of their product.
They add in salt and sugar and additives and flavourings to make you eat more and keep coming back for more.
Processed foods are literally *designed to be addictive*.
Designed.
Not a word that should be used about a 'food'.
It is hardly your fault you cannot stop eating those sweets.
A team of PhDs work to ensure that you don't!

The reason the dominant fizzy soft drinks taste better than a supermarket brand soft drink is because of the level of investment from their brand in creating the most addictive product available.

More nutrient dead 'food' goes in.
More calories, more malnourishment, more body fat, more hunger.
More money for the people selling it to you.

Supplements

Supplementation is sometimes seen as unnatural or unnecessary.
The first argument is laughable considering the 'food' that most people eat, and the second was covered above.
It is extremely hard to get a full complement of micronutrients – vitamins and minerals – from your food supply.
This is not a good place to be, but is unfortunately the reality of the situation.

Most people are aware of the Recommend Daily Amount (RDA) of vitamins and minerals as published by the government.
The RDA numbers are based on a population average, which doesn't really tell us much as we are all different; and it gives only the minimum amount you need to not get ill.
So, for example, the RDA of vitamin C is based on the amount you need to not get scurvy.
This is wildly different from the optimal level for health.
The RDA is the absolute bare minimum you should be eating.

Ideally, we would all get more nutrition, and if that necessitates the use of supplements then that is fine.
Really it's not possible to be 'too nutritioned' (that's not a real word…).
Yes, certain things are toxic in mega high doses and you should be careful, but that is no reason to shy away from them all together.
High quality products and qualified professionals have the knowledge and understanding to recommend a sensible dose *for better health*.

Your body doesn't recognise 'food' in the way your conscious mind does, it only recognises nutrition. If the nutrients you ingest are biologically the same and come from a natural source and not a laboratory, your body doesn't know any different.

This is why supplements can make a beneficial and easy addition to help a healthy diet.

If you drink vitamin C from orange juice or you eat a carrot, your body knows no difference between the two.

It is just vitamin C.

Exactly the same if you take a vitamin C supplement.

It is just vitamin C.

The body recognises macronutrients and micronutrients.

Proteins, fats and carbohydrates.

Vitamins and minerals.

It doesn't know what food you're eating or what form it comes in.

It just knows that you've ingested a certain amount of zinc, selenium or vitamin B6.

Supplementation needs can be very individual, dependent on your own very specific circumstances.

There are some basics that everybody will find safe and effective for improving their health and body.

We will cover only these basics and suggest that you see a specialist to go more in depth.

Quality in supplements is possibly even more important than in food.

Avoid high street brands that are dirt cheap.

Often they do not even have in them what it says on the label, or they do but it is not bio-available.

This means it is there, but in a form your body cannot absorb – pretty useless!

Use a high quality, pharmaceutical grade supplement.

It costs a bit more but it actually works, so it delivers value.

The cheap stuff is a waste of money.

Some of the brands that we recommend and are commonly available:

- Solgar

- Metagenics

- Biotics research

- Poliquin

- Eskimo oil (fish oil)

Vitamin D

We synthesise Vitamin D predominantly from sunlight and in the UK it is hard to get enough sunlight.
Everyone works indoors all day and there's not much sun here most of the year anyway.
In the past people worked outside more, in fields and the like.
Since the industrial revolution, people have shifted their lifestyle to being inside all day, making it tricky to get enough vitamin D.
Deficiency of vitamin D is mostly implicated in bone diseases such as rickets and osteoarthritis but study after study is showing it beneficial for general wellness and any number of other unrelated conditions.
Think of any illness or disease and there will probably be a connection to insufficient vitamin D, or evidence that optimal levels improve symptoms.
This is one supplement that everyone should consider taking.
We recommend you get tested; it's cheap and easy.
Ensure you know where you are at.
Do the test to make sure, but most people don't have nearly enough and benefit hugely from supplementation.

Digestive enzymes

For various reasons, people don't digest their food very well.
Other things aside (such as gut health), this is partly to do with stomach acid levels and partly enzyme production.
Stress is a big factor, be that mental stress, physical stress, illness, crap food – the body only knows stress, not its cause.
Stress represses stomach acid production.
People have a more stressful life than they used to in generations gone by.
It is an unfortunate fact of the modern world.
So everyone has less stomach acid, meaning they don't digest food as well, and don't extract sufficient nutrition from it.
If you eat food that has low nutrition anyway, and then you barely absorb what it does have, it's a lose/lose situation.
We recommend looking in to supplementing with a digestive enzyme.

Just a little bit could go a long way.

Your own natural production does start to come back after a while so it's not something you'll need to take forever.

You see the benefits very quickly when you begin to digest food, in reduced hunger, more energy and better hair, skin, nails etc.

Multivitamins

Multivitamins are generally a good bet for most people.

Even if you eat organic food, it's still difficult to get the full quota of all the vitamins and minerals you need.

A multivitamin is a quick, easy and cost effective way to fill in the gaps.

Magnesium and zinc

Most people have very low levels of these two minerals.

Magnesium has many benefits, including directly helping sleep patterns and digestive transit.

Spraying magnesium behind your knee before you go to bed will help you sleep.

Zinc is great for the immune system and skin and hair.

Supplementing with a bio available form of zinc may turn out to be the cheapest and healthiest beauty regime you could undertake.

They often come packaged together in supplements as 'ZMA'.

Evolution

Evolutionarily we are fundamentally the same as all other animals.

We may be more intelligent, but when it comes to eating, we don't know better than nature and we don't know better than other animals.

Frankly, our intelligence is becoming our downfall in this area.

We are too smart for our own good.

If you find a wild animal and try to feed it a donut, it probably won't eat it.

But give it a steak and it'll devour it (assuming it's a carnivorous animal of course).

Animals know what food is.

They haven't had the ability to manufacture anything different.

The concept that natural food that existed before we could manufacture it is somehow unhealthy for us is completely against the laws of evolution. We human beings can sometimes be exceptionally arrogant in our thinking.

In the grand scheme of human history, the human genome (our genetic make-up) doesn't change quickly.
Prior to mass manufacturing we couldn't make processed food, so we ate what was available from nature.
Real food.
We're not adapted to eating processed food or even to agriculture (read: grains).
When we first started harvesting wheat and sugar, the problems started.
We become afflicted with 'lifestyle' diseases.
When we started trying to control the natural environment and make our own food, everything went wrong.

Processed food correlates with lifestyle diseases such as diabetes, cancer and obesity.
Many 'foods' we are told to eat are not even edible!
Not until they are processed anyway.
So it's basically poisonous to begin with, then we process it into edible 'food'.
Seriously?
Wonder why people are no longer thriving?
Wonder why we are getting fatter year upon year?
Wonder why this is the first generation with lower life expectancy than the previous one?

It's not cyanide, but it is still poisonous to some degree.
Slowly but surely, it catches up with you.
It's like smoking; nobody ever contracted lung cancer from one cigarette.
'Food' that has to be processed to be eaten should not be eaten!
It is not food at all.

Our physiology is designed to deal with the food we're naturally supposed to eat.
Humans are omnivorous, which is why we can digest plants and animals.

We are not designed to digest grains properly.
We are certainly not designed to digest vegetable oils.
We are 100% not designed to digest 'Anti foaming agent polydimethylsiloxane'.

Yes, that is a real thing.
Used in medicine, cosmetics, some takeaway food, chicken nuggets and fries.

Physiology and food

We have adapted to certain tastes through evolution.
Generally, if it tastes bitter you won't like the taste of it because it's likely to be poisonous.
If it's sweet, it's safe to eat and energy-dense – a great coup.
When people stop eating processed food, they find that fruit and vegetables actually start to taste sweet.
You can taste the difference and the subtlety of different produce.
This is how people who live a healthy lifestyle survive without sugar and cakes.
They enjoy real food!

As most people are used to drinking 10 teaspons of sugar in one can of fizzy drink, they lose their sense of what sweet is.
Food manufacturers have taken advantage of our reactivity to sweet (and all tastes for that matter).
People crave foods that are sweet and salty, so they make things thousands of times sweeter and saltier than they would ever appear in nature.
Now your body craves even more of them.
As far as your body is concerned this is the Holy Grail.
It doesn't realise food is abundant and that you are getting fat and sick from over-consumption.
Hunter gatherer tribes, such as the Masai in Kenya, have their old wisdom.
They have known and learnt from thousands of generations.
Cut off from the western world and technology, they know exactly what to eat and what not to eat.
What is healing and what is poisonous.

There, and in places like Tibet, you find indigenous tribes that eat cows, drink their milk and blood and use the whole of the animal.
Whereas in the western world, people have a massive disconnect with where food comes from.
Many simply can't imagine where food comes from.
'It sounds disgusting!'

A lot of people can't even envisage raw food.
If it doesn't come nicely prepared as a meal, ready to open and eat, many consider it alien or disgusting.

Western scientific compartmentalisation

One of the predominant differences between western research versus say Chinese and Indian wisdom, is that we tend to look at things on their own.
We compartmentalise everything into single units and do not view the body and environment as holistic entities.
No one input can be responsible for an outcome.
No one outcome is the result of specific inputs.
The body is a system of systems.
Something can go wrong, and five levels down the chain a symptom may present in a totally different part of the body.
Something is wrong with your gut and you have depression.

Someone has cancer and they look for a miracle cancer drug.
This one pill will combat cancer.
The end.

All very logical and mechanistic sounding.
Shame it doesn't quite work like that.

You get ill for a reason.
One reason being what you put into your body.
As the old adage goes, 'prevention is better than cure'.
Prevent yourself from getting ill in the first place by not putting toxins into your body.
No one can argue that smoking doesn't cause cancer (except the tobacco companies), so like we said, it's not exactly far-fetched to consider that other toxins you put into your body cause cancer too.

'Everything in moderation' and 'a balanced diet' are BS

If you think about it logically, everything in moderation makes no sense at all.
Why put 50% crap in to your body to balance 50% valuable nutrition?
That is just dumb.

50% of the time I don't play in traffic…
So it's OK to go do it the other 50% of the time?
No!
You won't get any less run over!

Being healthy and looking after yourself some of the time doesn't justify eating unhealthy food the rest of the time.
It is just an excuse to eat junk food and a justification for not looking after yourself.
What are you trying to balance?

We don't want to come across as 'holier than thou'.
If you want to eat shit, that's cool.
Just don't kid yourself into saying you 'earned it' by caring about yourself earlier.

It comes down to values: how much do you value yourself and your health?
If you value yourself, you shouldn't see looking after yourself as a chore.

Unfortunately, food is marketed to encourage this hedonism.
'A little bit won't hurt.'
Many processed food manufacturers know their products are bad for you even in small quantities and have nothing good to say about them, so they get around this by seducing you into indulgence.
Pretty much the same strategy a drug dealer might use on an impressionable teen, no?
The only difference is, they manage to do it and remain socially acceptable!

A bit of sugar is not going to kill you.

Of course it won't.

But little quantities of wheat can do you harm. Depending on your reactivity.

Just cutting down to a small amount of wheat a day is pretty redundant.

You might as well just have a lot.

A lot of people have such a hard time accepting that they can't eat certain foods.

It's nonsensical to miss eating something you know is so bad for you.

Your emotions are ruling your logic.

Sometimes people like to do things that are bad for them… but it doesn't make it ok.

It is human nature, but you should discourage yourself.

Don't beat yourself up, though.

This never helps.

Realise the root of your problem and work to fix it.

There is not as much money to be made from selling people fruit and vegetables.

Multinational corporations don't advertise healthy fruit and vegetables because they can't make any money out of them.

They can and do make lots of money from selling you junk food.

Manufacturers want to make as much money as possible out of something that costs as little as possible, like vegetable oils.

Its basic business and you can't blame them in that sense.

Unfortunately, when you're playing with people's health, the morality is… questionable.

Learn to cook, love to cook

To drastically improve your health and your diet, all you need to do is cook from scratch.

Do this and you're most of the way there without even needing to be told what to eat or not eat.

It doesn't take as much time and effort as you might think.

Find time to cook and you will reap the benefits.

If you 'can't cook', learn how to cook and you will reap the benefits.
Follow a recipe, take a course, learn from friends/family…
This is not a viable excuse when it is so easy to overcome.
If you want to.

People value taste over their health, which is why people unconsciously opt for unhealthy food.
Most people who go on diets want to lose weight, but still want to eat junk food.
Not many actually want to stop eating fattening food.
This reflects their values and what they think about themselves.
They are junk food eaters.
It's how they identify with themselves.

Once people actually do commit to living a healthy lifestyle, most of them find it really easy.
When you commit fully to changing, it becomes easy.
Everyone can whip up meat and two veg.
If you claim you cannot, you are lying to yourself; the difficulty is purely mental and emotional.
You don't want to do it.
You don't want to believe that you can do it.

People should know how to look after themselves, but so few of us do.
This is not good enough!
We are passionate about changing this.

Do This: Read our recipe plans (Page 146)

- Start making tasty and healthy recipes today

Preparation is key

The key to a healthy lifestyle is good preparation.
To make sure you stick to your good intentions, once or twice a week go to the market and butchers and buy your fresh food.
If you don't have any, you're not going to make any.

If you have processed and unhealthy food in the house, you're going to eat processed and unhealthy food.

When you're feeling hungry and craving food, too much choice can be a bad thing.

You should have made the choice already when you went shopping and bought good food.

That way, when you're hungry or it's time to cook, you make what's there with the food available because that's what you've got.

You take the choice away when you're thinking straight.

Away from the irrational places known as hunger and cravings.

Everyone should have a selection of easy, go-to meals in the house.

These don't need to be processed, packaged or unhealthy.

Make your own 'ready meals'.

You can make simple curry, chilli, stew or casseroles: cook it at the weekends.

Make extra and freeze in portions so you can reheat throughout the week when you're too busy to cook.

If you come home from work tired, you can just reheat your healthy food.

You can take it to work for your lunch.

This way, you won't make unhealthy food choices and find yourself eating junk food.

It is much better for your health.

Plus it's cheaper, so you'll save some money.

Spend the money on quality of ingredients, rather than convenience.

There are also lots of quick and easy meals you can prepare yourself in minutes that are not unhealthy.

Stir fry is so quick and painless, all you need is a pack of vegetables and some prawns or meat and it takes about two minutes to prepare.

A healthy omelette only takes minutes.

As does steak and vegetables.

Your diet doesn't have to be gourmet cuisine; you can eat simple, healthy food at home without spending hours in the kitchen.

For people who say they have no time to cook…

You do.

We all have five minutes.
It takes that long to ping a microwave anyway, so why not opt for a healthy meal instead?

Embrace cooking.
Embrace the fact you're doing something good, being healthy, eating good food, and looking after yourself.
Once you accept the fact you are eating good food and that you are in it for the long run you will naturally start to focus on all the tasty foods you can have and forget about the stuff you cannot!

Most people would say a good steak is better than a sweaty oven pizza.
Good food is actually tastier!
The sooner you stop obsessing about what you can't have and focusing on all the positive aspects of embracing a healthier lifestyle, the sooner it becomes sustainable and easy.

Invest in some cookbooks and learn to make new, delicious and healthy food from scratch.
You might discover that you actually like a lot of food that you didn't think you would.
It may take a little while for your tastes and psychology to change, but it will happen, and you will reap the rewards both financially and physically.
You open your mind up to a whole new world.

Do This: Create a shopping list

- Based on the food guidelines and recipe book, create a shopping list for the week, to get all the ingredients you will need

- Set up food delivery if you feel that you do not have time to go to the shops for fresh food. Supermarkets do it, and a lot of great butchers and organic farms deliver high quality meat, eggs and produce straight to your door. Just Google 'organic meat delivery'.

- Whilst you're at it, throw away all of the crappy junk food you have in the cupboards if you are serious about not eating it anymore.

Ditch the deprivation mind-set

People often suffer from a feeling of deprivation.
Focused only on what you cannot have.
What is missing.
Always the negative.
If all you think about is what you can't have and how much you hate what you're doing, you're not going to be successful.
You will quit soon.
You're stuck in a negative deprivation mindset that is toxic.
Try to fight that with motivation and willpower and it won't last forever.
Before long you'll cave in and start eating junk food again.
The willpower never wins.

There is another way!
With no hunger and no deprivation.

CHECKLIST

Have you:
- ✓ **Downloaded the 'Eat this, not that' guidelines**
- ✓ **Downloaded the recipe e-book**
- ✓ **Used the recipe book and guidelines to plan meals for the coming week**
- ✓ **Created your shopping lists**
- ✓ **Organised food delivery (if applicable)**

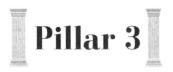

Pillar 3

Live a natural lifestyle

In conjunction with a healthy diet and exercise, lifestyle factors are vital components for good health.

Yet this is so often overlooked.

Not just by the general public, but also those in the fitness and healthcare communities.

Case Study: Lisa

Lisa was already a bit of a fitness bunny.

She was eating well and going to the gym four to five times a week.

But something was missing.

Progress had stagnated and she was frustrated with a lack of return from the effort she was putting in.

When she started to address some of her lifestyle factors, her fitness and strength went up, and she also got leaner.

Through a focus on consistent sleeping patterns, less alcohol and more recovery exercise, her strength and running times both improved for the first time in a while.

Altering some of the beauty products she used, along with an extra clean diet and some supplementation, allowed her to target the stubborn fat around the thighs where she tends to store fat.

As she turned 40 she was in the best shape of her life!

Stronger than ever, running quicker than ever and leaner than ever.

Nothing was added to what she was already doing – in fact she was encouraged to exercise less

It was just a few simple adjustments to her lifestyle that were very easy to implement.

THE MOST COMMON LIFESTYLE MISTAKES
YOU MAY HAVE MADE IN THE PAST

- Not managing stress.

- Always being busy and doing things for other people, but never prioritising making time for and looking after yourself.

- Using too many bad quality beauty products, adding to your toxic load.

- Not spending time playing or doing things just for the enjoyment of doing them.

- Not sleeping enough and having bad sleep hygiene.

---

30 SECOND TAKEAWAY TIPS

- This is not an all or nothing thing. Every single one of us can do things to improve our lifestyle and take action to being fitter and healthier.

- Managing stress is possibly the most important thing to deal with when you want to get healthier.

- Sleep quality is massive for its direct and indirect effect on health and resting should be given at least as much thought as working out.

- People nowadays spend far too little time relaxing and playing, or doing things just for the joy of doing them.

- The products you use on your skin, hair and body end up in the blood stream and if sourcing the highest quality is not prioritised can be a huge toxic burden on the body, causing general lower health, fat storage around the hips and thighs and cellulite.

- Prioritise yourself sometimes and make room to look after yourself. Managing your mental and physical wellbeing through relaxation, play and pampering.

When we want to get healthier, fitter, stronger or lose weight we tend to focus on diet and exercise in some combination, depending on our goals. We completely avoid even thinking about our lifestyle.

What do we mean when we say lifestyle factors?

The amount of sleep and sunlight we get, our stress levels, relaxation, happiness, play/fun and structured recovery.

Basically, lifestyle means everything that affects your body and your hormones that isn't diet or exercise.

Most people don't think about it and it's rarely talked about in the media.

It's easy to market a gym or a new diet, but no one makes money telling you to play more.

To be genuinely healthy it's vital to consider your whole lifestyle, not just how much exercise you do.

Manufacturers can't really sell more sleep or more daylight (if only).

There's no leverage, no incentive, so unfortunately it tends to get ignored.

Conventional western wisdom looks at health issues in separate, segmented parts and often ignores the lifestyle factors that cumulatively contribute to ill health.

There is actually a lot of research into how lifestyle factors affect hormonal balance and how this affects illness, health, weight etc, but it's not often taken into consideration or even acknowledged.

Lifestyle factors can be easy to change

On a personal level, lifestyle factors are sometimes the easiest and sometimes the hardest things to change.

You have control over whether you turn the lights and TV off at night.

It's much harder to control how much sleep you get with a new baby or how much daylight you get stuck in a dingy office.

If you work for 14 hours a day in a dark office, it's virtually impossible to get enough daylight.

But the barriers to change are more physical and practical rather than mental and emotional.
Nobody was every scared of letting go of bad sleep quality.
Everyone would want to sleep better or be less stressed.
This makes the things that are within your control very easy to change.
Focus on them.
Do what you can.

This stuff is not absolute.
You don't require an all or nothing approach.
One night of bad sleep will not kill you.

People sometimes get too carried away and think, because they can't get it absolutely perfect, there's no point in doing it at all.
But getting 50% of the way there, or just as much as is possible, is definitely preferable to not at all.
It is still 50% better!

Modern life is hectic

We are so used to modern living, working inside all day with lighting everywhere and TVs, computers and phones.
Many of us have no concept of nature.
We've forgotten what it feels like to rise and sleep with the sun.
Most city-dwellers have lost the connection with the planet and are disconnected from the natural elements.
It's easy to be nocturnal.
Up all night working away on the laptop…
Before the invention of electricity, people would go to bed when it was dark.
In winter you would semi-hibernate because it was dark and there was nothing you could do about it.
There were far fewer kinds of entertainment.
There were no 3D TVs. No Tablets. No smart phones.

Modern living is so frenetic and on the go, we rarely get periods of genuine relaxation.
We hardly ever just do absolutely nothing.

We never play (as adults), or go for a hike just because we feel like it.
With a career, a busy social life, and all the other distractions when we do
have 'down time', we never manage to switch off.

See the connection

The way it affects you is not always obvious or immediately apparent.
It is a fairly clear connection that if you eat more sugar and processed
food you will get fat.
But most people don't see the connection with their lifestyle.
It requires a little more understanding of hormones and the body's
systems.
As people are starting to have a greater understanding of this, it's
beginning to get looked at more, with more research done on sleep and
relaxation techniques.
Looking at how it affects other things within the body and many health
markers.

Quality over quantity (again)

Similar to diet, lifestyle factors are predominantly about quality.
Most people will see some form of light in their day-to-day lives…
But is it natural sunlight or artificial light?
Your body recognises the quality of sunlight and sends a cascade of
hormones.
Artificial lighting is on a different spectrum; your body doesn't recognise
it.
You don't get the same release of endorphins and serotonin, the vitamin
D synthesis.
It's about quality more than quantity.

In the same way as diet and exercise, we need the right lifestyle inputs,
based on our evolution.
You should think of it as the environmental impact on your health.
Your body reacts to a lot of environmental lifestyle factors.
Some you can control. Some you cannot.

Lifestyle factors

- Sleep quality and quantity

- Light and dark rhythms

- Sunlight

- Air and water quality

- Relaxation

- Play

- Emotional happiness

- Social connections

- Physical relaxation and treatments

Some of these things are harder to alter; you cannot control the air quality around you.
It is just important to acknowledge that it is a factor.
(Or move to the countryside or coast.)

The stress factor

If you take most animals out of their natural habitat, unless you are a trained zoologist they will most likely perish.
Even with adequate food, water and the obvious things the animals needs to survive, most creatures still end up dying pretty quickly.
From stress, isolation, shock, or any number of other reasons.
Humans are similar. We are sensitive creatures too.
The body reacts chemically to stressors and doesn't differentiate where they come from.
If we are put under stress, it is stressful for the body.

Regardless of what is stressing us out, the body chemically reacts exactly the same way.

For example, when your partner leaves you, you live off five hours sleep a night, or when you have the flu, it doesn't know the difference.
It's just stress and all manifests itself in the same way.
The same way as when you eat sugar and processed food or don't exercise.
It's all stressful for the body in the same way, and it can't tell exactly why you're stressed.

It just knows you are unhappy and not looking after either your physical or emotional wellbeing.
Some people gain or lose weight, get blemishes, or suffer from insomnia.
Some have digestive upset, get ill or depressed.
People react differently but they're all manifestations of the body being under too much stress for too long, in some form or other.

Hormonal cascades

Many hormones run on a circadian rhythm.
The natural daily fluctuation that cycles every 24 hours.
When that is out of sync, because you're not sleeping enough or not sleeping at the right times, the shift in your hormones is going to affect your energy, make you gain or lose weight, get ill, or get an increase in junk food cravings.
Many of us crave sugary or carb-laden food when we're tired or suffering from stress.
Trying to address diet without addressing these lifestyle factors is going to be a losing battle.
You're working against your body's biology.
Your cravings will beat your willpower.

What you should be doing...

Sleep in the dark, at night time, making sure your bedroom is absolutely pitch black.
Use black out blinds if you live in a brightly lit area and don't leave a light on in the hall.

Even the little standby light on many electrical implements can have an effect on your sleep quality.

When you sleep better, you don't need to sleep as much and when you're generally healthier and when you eat well and exercise, you sleep better.

By prioritising your sleep hygiene you can actually feel better and be healthier whilst having more free time, with more energy.

Sounds almost too good to be true…

Someone should make an infomercial about this!

Most of us can survive adequately on seven hours of sleep a night.

If you get bad quality sleep, that is when you need more of it.

Turn off the electrical stuff around you when sleeping.

Aside from the obvious phone buzzing at you from under the pillow waking you up…

The electromagnetic field put out by electronic equipment will affect your sleep quality.

Your brainwaves are electric and are easily affected.

You don't want electrical input keeping your brain active when it is trying to rest.

During the day it's vital that you get as much daylight as possible.

Your circadian rhythm recognises when it gets light and sets off the hormonal cascade, which tells you to wake up and start your day.

The stress hormone cortisol is intrinsically linked with your natural rhythm and should be high in the morning and drop to its lowest point in the evening.

It wakes you up when it's high, giving you energy for the day.

As it drops in the evening, your body slows down so you can relax and go to sleep.

Your body will be confused if you artificially raise it with a blaring alarm and triple espresso, and then never actually see any daylight.

Vitamin D is integral to pretty much everything the body does.

You synthesise it from the sun.

In 30 minutes of full sun exposure you can synthesise up to 20,000 IUs.

In hot countries obviously it's easy to get the adequate amount of sunlight quickly, but in the UK in wintertime, it's impossible.

It has to be direct sunlight and has to be of a certain strength.

We recommend you look in to supplementing Vitamin D to fill in the gaps.

Relating to daylight and vitamin D is the condition seasonal affective disorder.

A lot of people suffer from depression in winter.

Even if you're not diagnosed, it's not hard to see that everyone's happier when it's sunny and warm.

We are just more cheerful in the summertime.

This is also related to hormonal rhythms and your melatonin and serotonin levels.

Not getting the adequate combination of daylight and darkness can affect your hormonal balance.

Serotonin levels are linked to dopamine and to melatonin.

Melatonin is the sleep hormone and is also affected by the stress hormones.

Basically, if you don't go to bed when it's dark and wake up when it's light, you won't be as happy.

You can follow the chain of hormones to see why.

Literally, by turning the telly off at night and stopping looking at your phone you will be happier.

Physiologically and psychologically.

Playtime

Fun and 'play' time is another important aspect of leading a healthy and happy life.

Nowadays more people than ever are career-driven and life is all very serious.

People don't play enough or have fun enough.

As adults it's seen as a childish waste of time.

This is sad.

Just being – having fun and doing something to no end other than enjoying doing it – is a beautiful thing.

Try it.

It makes you happy, living in the now.

Relaxing and enjoying yourself is a massive stress release.

It can be anything from socialising to playing sport or enjoying something you're passionate about.

So long as you're doing something simply for the pleasure of it rather than for a necessary outcome – the opposite of work.

Most people do everything to earn money or survive.
People, as adults, don't do enough things just for the sheer pleasure of doing them.

Exercise is a good example.
Most people train for a specific outcome – to look a certain way, or to lose weight.
The most successful people train because they love training.
They enjoy the process and focus on the act of doing exercise instead of the outcome.
Lo and behold they get the best outcomes by default and enjoy doing it!

Relax

Whether it is structured relaxation or just natural, random relaxing it is important to find the time for it.
Structured relaxation such as massage, yoga, Pilates or meditation is great if you struggle to slow down and find the time.
You get the same effect getting a manicure, playing chess, or doing whatever it is that you find enjoyable and relaxing.
The release of stress is exactly the same as your body winds down, regardless of what the activity is.
Ten minutes of mindfulness is one of the most effective ways to release stress; check out www.getsomeheadspace.com for instructions.

You are achieving balance of the two sides of your nervous system.
Your yin and yang if you're into Chinese medicine.
The parasympathetic system is the 'fight or flight', which is how people spend most of their life.
Always on the go, on edge, busy doing stuff and stressing about things.
To be healthy and happy there needs to be more balance.
More time spent in the sympathetic nervous system.
Doing something you enjoy, just for the sake of it.
Emptying the mind of thoughts and focusing on the now.
Do whatever you do to relax and it keeps you less stressed.

Sleep

A good night's sleep is fundamental for long term health.
You can easily deal with a couple of bad nights, but chronic sleep deprivation is extremely bad for you.
You lose insulin sensitivity, your stress hormones get out of whack and your immune system weakens.
Many don't realise what negative affects our sleeping patterns can have on our body.

Good morning

Waking up to a blaring alarm clock that shocks you into consciousness is not a good way to start the day.
It's not especially enjoyable either!

There are different cycles of sleep.
Putting it as simply as possible, there are phases of deep and light sleep.
You're supposed to wake in a period of light sleep, which is why you feel terrible if you're woken suddenly from a deep sleep.
When you wake up half an hour before your alarm goes off and you feel really good, you were in light sleep and ready to wake up…
But you decide to press snooze and get a bit more sleep...
When you wake up again 30 minutes later you feel strangely exhausted.
It's because you're in a different phase of sleep.
You were back in deep sleep and not ready to wake up.
Moral of the story: if you wake up naturally, get up.
Sleep cycles last approximately 90 minutes.

To feel refreshed and ready to start the day, you want to wake up as naturally and gently as possible.
If you can wake up without an alarm, this is the best way to do it.
If you go to sleep and get up at the same time every day, you can train yourself and you'll start to wake up naturally before your alarm goes off.
Your body loves consistency.
A light alarm that gets progressively lighter to wake you is also a great alternative.
It wakes you up slowly and naturally, so it's a really easy way to get in sync with nature.

Physical relaxation

Making time to relax physically as well as mentally is important.
Slow and gentle exercise such as yoga and tai chi are great.
As is stretching, or getting a massage.
Sauna, steam room and other treatments are another option.
Even straight up pampering… facials, pedicures and the like are a great way to wind down, relax and feel good about yourself.

Meditation/Mindfulness

Meditation has kind of a bad reputation as being a bit 'hippy'.
We would agree that sitting with your legs crossed, 'ommmmm'-ing for hours on end is, but meditation comes in other forms.
It can be as short as a couple of minutes and can mean just being conscious of the now.
Emptying your mind of thoughts and focusing on something, maybe the sound of the train on the tracks during your commute, or the feeling of your feet on the floor as you sit at the desk.
Forget about the worries for a moment and become present.
This can be an enlightening experience that some people will dismiss without trying.
Try it!

It is a great way to take a quick time out from the day.
De-stress and come back better.
Happier and more productive.
Just take a walk around the block and focus on counting each step.
It really is not hard.
So worth it, though.

Products

Anything you put onto your body ends up inside your body.
Shampoo, soap, moisturiser and make up actually absorb quicker through your skin than food does through your mouth.
It hits the bloodstream quickly as it doesn't need to go through your stomach for digestion.
So this stuff ends up in your body.

Ask yourself, would you eat this?

Obviously, not literally.

Nobody wants to chew on soap.

But if you did, would it be dangerous?

Is it poisonous?

That's not to say you can never put anything on your body that you wouldn't eat, but it's a good barometer.

Whenever possible, opt for natural products.

Organic skincare and other products are best.

Use the minimum dose you need.

It helps keep the toxic load down and the body healthy and functioning well.

There are so many toxins in a lot of the products that people use.

If you store fat around the thighs this is especially relevant for you, because the chemicals in products mimic estrogen in the body and an inability to sufficiently detoxify estrogens leads to storing fat on the thighs and upper arms.

Read the ingredients list and clock how many words you can pronounce…

You are looking to avoid parabens, xenoestrogens and BPA, first and foremost.

Check the ingredients of your products.

Detoxification - get rid of cellulite

Cellulite is a tricky subject for many people.

Not knowing why it is there, or how to get rid of it.

Even when you're lean, cellulite can remain.

Target cellulite by working on improving your detoxification pathways.

Drink a lot of water (3 litres a day), use saunas, exercise and supplement.

There are very specific supplements that can help with detoxification, and the removal of cellulite.

Detoxification is a complex subject that is beyond the scope of this book, but focusing on avoiding the toxins, and the point mentioned above is a good place to start.

What to do and how to do it

Make small changes to your lifestyle.

You can make one step at a time, and accumulate lots of small wins.

Because there's not any emotional connection or craving it's easier to change lifestyle factors.

Everyone can do one or two small things, which is not going to affect your life in any conscious way, but is going to be better for you.

Keep doing that and it builds up; you don't notice, but you're slowly getting better, healthier and more in sync with where you want to be.

You don't need to become obsessive about it.

People tend to get obsessive about diet and exercise, then burn out quickly, fail and give up.

As there's nothing overwhelming about small simple lifestyle changes based on logic it shouldn't be hard to maintain them.

Obviously, there are going to be certain aspects of your life that you can't control, but it doesn't have to be 100%.

It would be rather difficult to live in a cave without electricity.

But small adjustments will make big improvements to your health and wellbeing.

Simple adjustments like relaxing by candlelight, not having every light in the house on, switching off your TV and laptop, stretching or having a relaxing bath will switch off overactive brain activity so the stresses of the day start to go away and you'll sleep much better for it.

It's not hard to do, and you're not losing anything by doing it.

It is only positives.

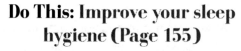

Do This: Improve your sleep hygiene (Page 155)

- Ensure you have a totally dark room, with blackout blinds if necessary

- Turn off all electronics before going to sleep

- Be consistent in your sleep pattern

- Wake up gently by investing in a light alarm

- Relax for 10 minutes before going to bed: stretch, have a bath, meditate or listen to relaxing music

Do This: Book a relaxing or restorative session at least once a month

- This can be yoga or tai chi, a massage or beauty treatment or guided meditation

- Concentrate on yourself and use these modalities to de-stress on a regular basis

Do This: Where possible swop beauty products for natural alternatives (Page 167)

- Look at how many products you use and shop around for healthier alternatives

- Try things out, see which natural alternatives suit you; some may not.

CHECKLIST

Have you:
- ✓ **Improved your sleep hygiene**
- ✓ **Booked a restorative session**
- ✓ **Made time to relax and play**

Pillar 4

Working out can and should be fun

When you enjoy something you keep doing it.
If you enjoy your training it becomes part of your life, part of your normal habits and something you want to do.
Eventually it becomes an intrinsic aspect of your lifestyle.
You will start to identify yourself as someone who works out.
It is now part of your day to day.

Case Study: Katherine

When Katherine came to us she was training for her first London marathon attempt.

She had the running thing down, but was not doing the strength and mobility work that makes you a more efficient runner and keeps you injury-proofed.

She had a target of four hours or under and was very determined to do it. Once she got into the training sessions and started having fun challenging herself, she found that she set and met a number of milestones along the way.

She did her first full press ups, and then added reps.

She learnt full squats, how to climb monkey bars and is well on the way to her first pull up and single leg squats.

Unfortunately, she narrowly missed out on the 4-hour marathon, but has since set a sub 50-minute 10k and completed the Tough Guy obstacle race, with another marathon in the pipeline very soon to go for that sub 4-hour time.

Katherine exemplifies someone who is determined and progressive in their training, setting and meeting a goal before moving on to the next one.

Making it an enjoyable and satisfying part of her life. Just as it should be.

THE TOP EXERCISE MISTAKES YOU MAY HAVE MADE IN THE PAST

- Too much cardio and neglecting strength training.

- Being inconsistent and losing interest for a period before returning to 'start again'.

- Doing things you dislike and seeing them as a chore, so hating every second.

- Not following a progressive plan.

- Neglecting having fun and socialising through exercise.

- Being stuck in a paradigm that defines exercise as the treadmill and doesn't consider fun activities and sports as great ways to enjoy exercise.

---

30 SECOND TAKEAWAY TIPS

- Doing challenging workouts consistently is the only way to progress and get better.

- Find something that you enjoy doing, something that inspires you and you will look forward to doing. This will allow you to actually sustain it.

- Prioritise strength training and relaxing exercise such as yoga. Then do one or two interval cardio training sessions per week if you want.

- Make working out fun and social: find a group of people, class, team or buddy to work out with. The social aspect is as important as the exercise when it comes to enjoyment and the likelihood that you will continue doing it.

- Look after mobility (flexibility through movement) and work to function and move well, before going hardcore with training. It stops you getting injured and makes you perform better.

You get into it and it starts being fun.
You start looking for new challenges and look to achieve something bigger.
As you make progress, you will inevitably start to push yourself.
It moves away from wanting to get healthier or lose weight or whatever reason you started.
You enjoy the process. Enjoy the doing.
Chase after achievement.
This is when you get great outcomes.
Funnily enough you reach a level where you forget about and almost stop caring about these original outcomes!
You're *that* person who loves exercise.
To whom it comes naturally.

Happy happy

Everyone feels good after a workout.
When you work out you release endorphins and lower stress.
It's impossible not to feel happy when you're brimming with happy hormones.
When you exercise regularly you get into this cycle of being happy.
Who doesn't want to be happy?

This good feeling will permeate the rest of your life and make you feel better, all the time.
You'll have more energy.
Your concentration and productivity at work will improve.
Your family life may improve.
Your zest for life goes up.
Everything may start to feel like it is running better.

You're pushing yourself.
Setting goals, finding your limits.
People love winning and achieving things.

They crave this feeling.
The biggest sense of achievement you can get is when you do something you didn't think you were capable of.
Something you previously thought was impossible.

Sense of achievement

It's a short- and long term sense of achievement.
The process of exercise, running further, lifting more, whatever it is, in the moment is a huge sense of achievement…
Then the bigger outcome: when you feel yourself change, your outlook changes.
You achieve a bigger long-term goal.
You have worked for something for a long time and made it.
It's a permanent sense of achievement.

You can feel yourself changing.
You feel fitter, all the time.
Walking up the stairs or running for a bus, everything becomes easier, more manageable.
You feel good daily.

Psychologically it's great for your confidence.
You will get to know yourself better and what your capabilities are.
You will experience pushing yourself, stretching to achieve something.
We all need to be achieving things, pushing ourselves both mentally and physically to feel happy.
You find your true self at the edge of your comfort zone.

For long-term health, exercise of course is beneficial and not just for the obvious reasons.
For example: being strong is vital for injury prevention.
When you are working out regularly , you're less likely to get injured in your day-to-day life if you're stronger.
You will have better balance, bone density, coordination, body awareness and you may even live a longer and healthier life.

This also leads to better performance in any sports that you do.
Strength training especially.

If you're a runner and you lift some weights, you'll be a better runner, get injured less and be more efficient.

Dislike exercise?
Working out doesn't necessarily have to involve treadmills and sweaty gyms.
People automatically think of endless trudging along on a treadmill when you say working out.
We hate this.
Probably so do you.
It is very boring and gives exercise a bad name!

Do something you love.
Something that you are passionate about.
Something that drives you to achievement.
Something that inspires you.
It doesn't matter what it is, if you're moving and working up a bit of a sweat it is going to be better for you than sitting on the sofa!
People who 'don't like' exercise automatically go to the treadmill.
Thinking only of the far off outcome they want.
They force themselves to do something they do not want to do.
Assuming that this is the only way.
This treadmill paradigm is funny…
Frankly, it isn't a very effective way to exercise, even if you do manage to stick with it!
Try something new: try a sport, try a competition, try something with a team or with friends.
Partaking in a sporting activity that you enjoy doing is better for your motivation and your enjoyment.
By challenging yourself and having new experiences, you'll grow as a person.

People need to stray from their default setting to find out what works for them.
Take risks in life.
Dare to ask questions and find out the answer.
Try something different.

Escape from reality.
In the moment, get your teeth into the process of what you are doing.
Take time out from your normal work day and empty your mind.
Be in almost a meditative place when exercising.

Make your training schedule a social event.
There are lots of different options, including gym classes, boot camps, running clubs and sports teams.
Train with other people, get a gym buddy, work with a professional, or meet people at the gym or wherever you wish to train.

By exercising with friends you are creating accountability as you make a commitment to another person as well as to exercise.
When it's a group, it's social and fun but you also don't want to let your teammates down.
Whether that is an actual team, or just your 'team' of Saturday morning jogging buddies.

Trying a new type of exercise is also a great way to meet people and make new friends.
Try new things and do different things together.
Meet new people and you get a different perspective.
Meeting new people has many other benefits beyond the actual exercise process.
Business connections, friendships, a support network.
You can forget about the exercising and see it as a way to build social connections and networking if it makes you enjoy it more!

Generally, everyone's in the same boat.
You can become part of a group where you all come to the same place to do the same thing.
Your goals and motivations are aligned.
Your friends will have empathy.
Everyone's been through or is going through the same thing as you.
Everyone can relate to one another.
This collective identity really connects people.
You feel part of the group.

It's a basic human need to feel wanted and to be part of something, such as a tribe or a movement.

Nobody gets left behind in a group.
When you train alone it's very easy to lose motivation and give up.
With a group identity you encourage each other, and help drive each other forwards.
It feels good to help other people.
They feel good and it makes you feel good too.
If you're more experienced, motivating and helping others is good for everyone.
Obviously it helps them and it reinforces what you have learnt and drives you on.
A collective sense of 'us against the challenge', being in it together against the run, the workout or the challenge.

Laugh.
Try and laugh during every group training session.
Enjoy yourself.
If you're enjoying it and having fun you look forward to it.
You want to go because it is fun!

Friendly competition will drive you on, drive progress.
Time flies when you're having fun and it suddenly won't feel like a chore.
A lot of people who 'dislike exercise' get into the group, have fun and enjoy the experience.
This brings results, because you stick with it…
And consistency is king.
Even if you still 'dislike' exercise, unless you're an athlete it doesn't need to be serious!
Have fun with it, detach from the outcome obsession and enjoy it.

The 30-minute workout

You really don't need to spend ages working out.
You can do just half-hour training sessions and see all the benefits you want.
It's easy to fit it in, in the morning, at lunch or after work.

Thirty minutes is not a massive commitment of time, but it's plenty to make a huge difference to your fitness.

You can achieve just as much with half an hour of intensive exercise as you would in three times as much time spent half-arsing it.
You get a better workout in less time by putting some intensity in to it.

Thirty minutes is enough to achieve long term results.
A little, often and consistently: half an hour once a day.

Training for longer is not necessarily a bad idea, but the point is that you don't *have* to.
If you're busy and struggle fitting it in or don't want to commit any more time.
Just find 30 minutes, three times a week.
Not having enough time is not a good excuse.
Make time!
As long as you work hard in the time that you do have, it's fine.
Thirty minutes fits in your life easily.
You don't need to feel overwhelmed or like you spend your whole life in the gym.

You can train anywhere in the world.
The gym obviously has better equipment, but doing anything is better than nothing.
You can work out at home or in the park, in the garden, or even your hotel room.
You've got no excuses, so use what's around you.

Being in the gym and using weights is preferable. But training on the living room floor is still better than lying on the sofa.
Do what you can.
Make sure you start at the level you're at.
Don't try to do too much if you have never worked out before.
At this stage, anything will work.
As you progress you need to be more structured and more intense.
Keep it fun, you don't need to get too obsessive with it.
Keep progressing and trying to do a bit more.

Work a bit harder.
Keep chipping away.

Different types of training

Fundamentally, people need to be lifting heavy weights in big movements.
Using lots of muscles and lots of joints.
You will see lots of examples in the workout plans coming up shortly.
Try and use the heaviest weights that you are comfortable with.
Not too comfortable, mind…you need to push yourself.

It's the most effective way to get fit and has the biggest effect on your body.
It is also the most efficient use of time.
You don't need to train 84 different muscle groups.
Five or six big simple exercises will be enough.
Squats, dead lifts, presses, pulls, rows, carries and some sort of abs and core.
A few primary movement patterns and you hit all the right muscles.
The big exercises will have the greatest effect on your hormones and the biggest energy boosting capacity.

The benefits of lifting weights and getting stronger include:

- Injury prevention

- Functional every day strength

- Ability to lift things and pull things

- Strength carries over to other sports/activities and general life

- Increased bone density

- Avoiding muscle atrophy (shrinking)

- Stress relief

- Good release of aggression

- Building confidence

- Releasing 'feel good' hormones

- Fat loss

- Hormonal balance

- Increase in lean tissue

- Burn more calories

- Resting metabolic rate increases (meaning your metabolism is permanently faster, and you burn more calories)

There's no difference in how you should train for weight loss, toning, strength or fitness.
There are parameters you should modify but essentially it's the same.
Only when you get in to the realms of performance do things get a little more intricate.
Whether you wish to get stronger or lose weight, the training is still essentially the same.
The diet is driving the different outcome.

Indeed, there is no difference when people talk about losing weight or toning.
It is exactly the same thing.
'Waste yourself away doing cardio, to lose weight, and then do weights to tone up' is a fundamental misunderstanding of how the body works.
Tone means better muscle definition, with less fat.
You don't lose weight and then get toned; it's all the same thing.
You appear 'toned' by losing weight and building muscle…
And building muscle helps you lose weight.

You don't want to be skinny fat.

This is where you are very light in bodyweight, but still carrying too much fat.

Usually achieved through lots of cardio and caloric restriction.

Though some people who have a fast metabolism and are genetically slim can do it simply by eating crap and not training.

Look at sprinters and other power athletes, they are lean and look great.

Think Jessica Ennis and Victoria Pendleton.

A lot of amateur distance athletes are very thin but still flabby.

Make sure, if you are in to endurance sports, you are working on strength and eating enough too.

Weights for the girls

Unfortunately, many women feel intimidated by the idea of lifting weights.

If this is you, please do not worry.

Most men don't know what they're doing any more than you.

And indeed are much less likely to take advice or help.

Obviously you want to feel comfortable whilst pushing yourself and training hard.

If you're not there yet, try not to feel nervous about going into the weights room in your gym.

Everybody started somewhere and most people empathise with beginners.

The chances are, anybody in there will respect you for making that step, rather than looking down their nose at you.

Don't be afraid to put some effort in and train hard.

Don't be averse to sweat.

Nobody cares when you're at the gym.

Especially if you're with a group of other women also training hard.

These days, 98% of personal trainers make women lift weights.

Simply because it works.

This is helping it to become more socially acceptable.

Educating and empowering more women to be able to train alone or teach their friends.

Just as it should be.

You only need look at the outcomes for proof.

Go to a gym, look at everyone on the treadmills and most of them will be out of shape.

Then look at everyone in the weights rooms and the majority of them will be lean and fit.

It's not a coincidence.

It's because they are training right!

Feminine values are starting to change.

Women traditionally didn't work to be strong.

But now 'strong is the new skinny', is a reflection of society's values.

Of course, we think strong was always sexy.

But it seems the unhealthy size zero look is out and lean and toned is in.

Medical professionals used to actually say lifting weights was bad for women.

Until recently women weren't even legally allowed to enter marathons.

This was based on… absolutely zero evidence.

Perhaps just a reflection of what society – or the people in power – wanted to portray.

Thankfully, advances in scientific evidence and public opinion have changed all this.

It is acceptable for women to look and be strong and people are gaining awareness of how important it is for health as well as just wanting to feel toned and athletic.

However, there is still a lack of accessible information specifically available to women.

Sounds silly in the internet era when you can find any information about anything.

Of course it is out there.

But not in a concise and simple way, without someone trying to sell you the latest wobbly board or shake diet.

Most of the information surrounding strength training is aimed at men, with a focus on body building.

Whilst it isn't wholly different, there are considerations relating to the differing hormonal profiles of men and women.

As far as women are concerned, aerobics DVDs are the most popular and

readily available resource.
These greatly underestimate women's potential…
And are a bit of a scam.

One of the problems is that many women feel more comfortable doing cardio.
So they default to it.
Partly because they've never had access to decent information that states otherwise.
They assume this is what they should be doing.

To see results you need to get away from just doing what you have always done and experiment with training.
Women need to do more weights, more mobility work (dynamic flexibility through movement) and less slow and repetitive trudging on the treadmill.

Mobility

Sitting at a desk all day is bad for your mobility (unsurprisingly) and can lead to chronic injury including bad backs, ITB-itis (scientific term), neck ache, sore knees etc.
A combination of stretching, manual therapy (osteopathy, chiropractic, massage, ART, physiotherapy) and self-release (explained below) should give you a sufficient range of motion in your joints, which will lead to better athletic performance, less chance of injury, less chance of chronic discomfort, better posture, better breathing and being more awesome!

Do it yourself

You can do stretching and self-release yourself.
Self-release is essentially achieving the same as a massage, but doing it yourself.
You may have seen a 'foam roller' in your gym, the foam tube.
Rolling the length of the muscle over the roller creates a release of tension.
Less tension means more flexibility or mobility.
All is demonstrated below.

**Do This: Download the mobility program
(Page 181 and www.aretefitness.co.uk/mobility/)**

- Work on at least one area of mobility for at least five minutes every day, first thing or before bed.

- Once a week spend 30 minutes dedicating time to mobilising.

And relax

On top of the getting strong and mobile we also recommend some relaxing low impact exercise.
Like tai chi, yoga or a type of martial art.
It is as much mental as physical.
De-stressing and slow moving to balance the 'aggressive' strength training.
Yoga for example is something you can do at home with a DVD, very easily.
You will feel so much better for it and can use it in the evenings to wind down before bed.

Cardio

We're not dismissing cardio completely.
It is beneficial in sensible doses.
It's better to do short sharp intervals rather than continuous cardio.
30 minutes at a time.

**Do this: Download our interval
training program (Page 181)**

- Do the interval training program once or twice per week.

- The priority is intensity. Work as hard as you can!

Obviously, if you're training for a marathon you'll need to do more. But for general health or fat loss, intervals are quick and effective and you won't need to do them more than twice a week.

Do This: Download our complete strength training program (Page 181)

- Go to www.aretefitness.co.uk/exercises for full video demonstration of all of the exercises

- Do the strength training program two to three times a week.

- Find a gym buddy to train with if you need some motivation and help working out.

Don't forget to go to the website www.aretefitness.co.uk to gain access to all the free resources above.

CHECKLIST

Have you:
- ✓ **Downloaded the mobility program and found five minutes daily to undertake it**
- ✓ **Downloaded the training calendar and scheduled your sessions into your diary**
- ✓ **Downloaded the interval training program**
- ✓ **Downloaded the strength training program and watched the videos to learn the exercises**

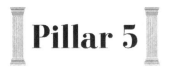

Pillar 5

Make positive habits to break negative habits

In many ways, this final pillar is the culmination of the other four.
Creating the right habits is the fundamental piece in your health and fitness jigsaw.
It is a habit that makes for long term, sustainable, 'easy' results.

Get the habit

Everything we do, whether right or wrong, is a habit, unless you make a sustained, conscious effort to change it.
A habit is stronger than your willpower and habits will always win eventually, because they are imbedded in your subconscious mind.

This is not a reflection of your weakness, or some character flaw.
It is simply the way it is.
Those who are 'more successful' are not stronger than you, they are better prepared.
Often they do not know it themselves, but they are able to 'do the right thing' – hit the gym, avoid the donut, quit smoking – because they have a support structure in place that allows them to.
Habits are your brain's way of taking shortcuts on an unconscious level.

Case Study: Orsi

Orsi is possibly the best example of preparation and process becoming habit that we know.

She is highly motivated, due to managing some health issues that make straying off track very uncomfortable and really just not worth it at all.

Upon starting to make the changes to her life – eating (religiously) well, working out, quitting smoking and managing stress – it all seemed very daunting and overwhelming.

To overcome this she took one day at a time, addressing what needed to be done that day and nothing more.

As the days passed, her actions accumulated and the results became evident. Through consistently setting and meeting daily process goals, Orsi was able to completely turn her health and her life around.

Things that she thought she would miss – food and especially smoking – she just doesn't.

She has broken the old habits and created new positive habits that are aligned with her goals.

Not having junk food in the house, planning meals in advance and doing preparation work like batch cooking at the weekends.

Getting up early before work to go work out, and going to bed earlier to facilitate this.

Managing her stress levels and not taking on the world's problems along with her own.

All of these shifts have allowed Orsi to take control of her health and live a happier life.

Now she is much healthier, a fully-fledged exercise lover and running nut and all around a bit of a health freak.

Almost the complete opposite to how she was just 18 months ago.

Through making the right habits and attaining daily process goals, anything is possible.

THE MOST COMMON HABITS MISTAKES YOU MAY HAVE MADE IN THE PAST

- Not realising that most of what you do is out of habit.

- Not having process goals that aim to create the right habits in your life.

- Not keeping records and learning about yourself in order to structure a plan that is uniquely effective for your own circumstances.

- Trying to rely on your willpower to do the right thing.

- Being stop-start and never giving a good go of something before writing it off as ineffective.

30-SECOND TAKE-AWAY TIPS

- Set goals and prepare first, then base your plan on how you are going to achieve these through a number of defined daily processes.

- Know what processes you need to perfect to achieve your aim and how you will measure them, then implement, measure and tweak as appropriate. You need to perfect your plan, not give up or start afresh repeatedly.

- Understand your current habits through logging and observation, then create new positive habits to break the old negative habits. You will never stop doing something until you consciously create an alternative option.

- Avoid willpower by never being in a situation in which it is needed; a good plan and habits will achieve this. Relying on willpower guarantees that you will fail.

- Accumulate little wins to achieve grand scale success. It can seem an awful long way off, so breaking it down in to smaller pieces and rewarding things that are 100% in your control – the process goals – is the way to keep you progressing over the long term, until you achieve your big goals.

- Be consistent in your implementation, always. Tweak your plan to make minor improvements, but it is the consistent application of the basics that brings 90% of the progress. Just keep plugging away until you are where you want to be.

Most of your daily actions occur automatically.
You wouldn't want to have to do everything consciously, because then you would never get anything done.
Imagine consciously having to remember to walk or to breathe.
If your brain had to think about everything in a conscious way, you would be massively overloaded and likely curl up in the corner, a shivering, nervous wreck.
So, of course, it is natural for most of your daily actions to become habits to spare your poor neurons from burning out and smoke expelling from your ears (not a good look in the office).

Prepare First

As in Pillar One, set your goals first.
Then create a plan based on the goal.
The plan you devised earlier should now be implemented as a set of habits you are going to create in order to achieve your goal.
Create some accountability, so people know what you are doing and expect you to achieve something.
Tell your friends and family.
Tell them that you are going to achieve [your goal] and that you will be doing [your habits] to do so. This is a great motivational tool, especially if you tell people whose opinion you value.
You'll then want to live up to their expectations of you.
Nobody likes to disappoint.
Dig out the accountability sheet from earlier and add in some habits when you have finished reading this chapter.

If you do not have a goal and then a plan based upon it, if you just have a plan and no end goal, you never know if you're achieving anything or actually making progress.
Or fundamentally if what you are doing is right or wrong.
You must know this information and reassess regularly.

You need a goal, but also a structure of how to get from where you are now to where you want to be.
The structure tells you what you can or can't do.
Say you want to be a millionaire.
If you don't have a plan, you're just dreaming.
You need to know your destination first, but then you need to work out *how* to make a million.
Once you have your goal, work backwards on how to achieve it.

How many people have started the latest diet craze or the January Gym-athon to 'lose some weight'?
What on earth does that mean?!
Don't eat for a week and you will 'lose some weight'…
Are you any better off? No.
Are you any leaner? No.
Are you going to maintain this? No.
Are you healthier than before? No.
Was this a redundant exercise that took you further away from what you truly want? Yes.

You cannot make a plan without knowing, in detail what you want to get out of it!

Know What Processes You Must Achieve And How to Measure Them

Once you've got a plan then you must make sure all the effort you are putting in is productive and going in the right direction, so that you're not wasting your time or contradicting yourself.
Don't worry about chasing perfection.
Just make sure you have an outline or a structure of what you want to do.
Then start doing it.

You don't need information overload or to learn everything that was ever said about a subject. Just find something simple, that's going to work for you and logically makes sense and then start doing it.

This is the time for action.

The time to get shit done.

The time for reflection and questioning comes *after* you have started.

When you have some data to work with.

Make a plan but don't get caught up in lots of thinking and no doing.

Results, good or bad, only come from doing something.

If you don't do anything then you're not going to get any results.

If you have already started, you can tweak, but if you have not got round to doing anything then you will never get anywhere.

The point of making a structured plan and making it a habit…

You're not leaving it to chance; you're defining where you're going and how you are going to get there.

Imagine you are driving somewhere: if you know where you are driving to it's much easier to figure out the best route to take.

If you take a wrong turn, you can reassess and alter your journey.

But if you sit at home worrying, playing through in your mind a number of *disastrous* wrong turns and potential outcomes and never actually leave your house, you will never get anywhere!

Leave your house.

Good, now that you are on the road it is important to make sure you are not speeding off too fast. When you leave it to chance, you can get too highly motivated and rush off trying to do everything without actually thinking about it or planning.

You need to make a plan.

If you don't have a plan you're completely reliant on willpower and outside factors; without an underlying structure, a framework to refer back to, you just do *things*.

You end up wearing yourself out.

You have nothing to refer back to, in order to decide if you're on the right path.

Doing 'things' is often no more more use than doing nothing.

Say a situation arises, such as friends ask you out for pizza.
When you have a plan you can refer back to it and assess whether or not this will impact on your outcomes.
Otherwise you leave it to chance, and the chance of you falling completely off the fitness wagon is strong.
You get yourself in to a situation where you are doing things right or wrong, it is black or white, good or evil.
This is a dangerous place to get yourself and, for the sake of your self-esteem, you do not want to define yourself wholly by the latest choice you made...
Especially when you have nothing in place to ensure it was a good one!
If you have a plan, then you think: can I afford to have a bit of pizza?
Yes I can.
One pizza won't upset the whole cart.
Great.
Or: no, I shouldn't have pizza, it will set me too far back.
I shall go, but ensure I choose a meat dish instead.
Great.

Do This: Set your process goals (Page 139)

- Download the goal-setting sheet and set weekly process goals to achieve

- Keep the goals somewhere you will see and regularly update

Measuring outcomes is discussed in Pillar 1; you should also be measuring the processes and habits. When you have identified what you need to do in order to achieve your goal, this should become your focus, because this is what is within your control.
Do not define success solely by an outcome, because that is not within your control.
Of course, track it.
Of course it should be moving in the right direction.
Track the processes and habits, then you can alter them if need be, to improve the outcome.
Tweak, rather than reinventing.

If you have identified that often you miss training sessions because you get stuck in the office late in the evening, this is where you create a process that allows the solution to become a habit.

Train three times a week in the morning before work.

Measure it and make sure you are achieving it.

After a while it will become a habit – normal – and you will do it on autopilot.

Missing sessions?

No.

Problem solved.

If you had approached this same problem as, 'I don't train enough so will not improve my marathon time', and you just beat yourself up about missing sessions.

Helplessly blamed work and held a lot of negative feelings toward your job…

Do you think:

a) The problem would be solved?

b) You would make any progress on a personal level?

No, and No.

Channel energy in to leveraging what is in your control to work for you.

Log And Learn

You need structure so you can make progress.

Your plan should always be progressive. It avoids overwhelming yourself.

Some people will just change their life because they're planning for a wedding or an important event and it becomes part of their lifestyle, but generally if you don't have something to strive for, you'll find it difficult to sustain one huge wholesale change.

It shouldn't feel like you're doing too much, if the plan is affecting your whole life, then you're not going to do it very long and will quickly give up.

Lots of small wins will build confidence.

Break it down and make it seem more achievable and manageable.

Write down your processes and record the outcomes: this could be a food diary, workout log or daily journal.

You are collecting data, and data is the most valuable thing in your journey.

You are empowered by data.

Data gives you a base to compare your results against.

You can learn what works for you and what does not.

You remain accountable to yourself, and cannot reason away a failure unless it is justified.

You can measure your compliance and determine whether the plan you are following doesn't work, or whether, in fact, you are not actually following it.

If that is the case, there is either a problem with your plan or your mindset.

If it is too hard and unrealistic, you need to taper it back to something manageable.

Some progress is better than no progress!

If the plan looks achievable and you are simply not following it, you need to assess your values and goals, and then look at your day-to-day implementation, to work out where it is going wrong. Keeping logs and having data empowers you to do this.

Or you could just blame yourself.

Admit you are a failure and a bad person, and just give in.

Either way…

(You're not a bad person)

The reason you're not a bad person is because you are probably not going wrong on purpose.

It is probably because there is a habit you have not realised, or failed to plan for.

You will always revert back to what you know unless you do something to avoid it.

The only way to break an old habit is to create a new, better, super powered habit.

Habits are so engrained it's not worth the misery of *trying to stop*.

Instead *start doing something else instead*.

Make a positive habit to break a negative habit.

Do this instead of that.

Your brain will thank you for working with it instead of against it.

Your alarm clock goes off in the morning and you get up, you're hungry, and this signals time to eat.

No problem.

You're sad or stressed out and this signals it is time to eat.

Problem.

This is a bad stimulus-response.

This will have a bad outcome.

You want to break those habits more than anything else.

Most of your daily routine is identical, day in, day out, 95% of what you do, every day, is exactly the same.

Disruption is not well tolerated as your brain has to expend energy and think about it.

We are very much creatures of habit.

Changing requires thought.

If you go to a restaurant and don't think about it, you'll most likely go back to what you normally have.

But if you consciously scan the menu and think about what is the right thing to eat, which food is in line with your goals, you put thought into the process to alter the chain of habit, to stop you repeating your bad habits such as eating pizza 'because' you're at an Italian restaurant.

But it needs to be a conscious decision, so you need to be mindful of certain habits and attempt to change them by being aware of them.

Become mindful of your habits then you can strive to create better ones.

When you feel stressed or sad, try 10 minutes of meditation instead.

Maybe a walk around the block.

Whatever works for you.

When you go to the restaurant, get in the habit of reading the menu fully before deciding what you will have.

By slowing down and engaging your brain you will naturally become aware of what is going to be good or bad for your goals, and be empowered to make the right choice.

Avoid Willpower

Habits are easy to make but hard to break, so try replacing old habits with new healthy ones.
It's initially hard to go against your natural urge, so make sure you always line up alternatives.
Create good habits to alter bad ones.
If you're feeling deprived you'll never achieve anything.
By creating good habits, you're focusing on the positive of what you are doing.
When you have a plan you usually end up falling into a habit without realising it.
If you say 'my plan is to go to the gym three times this week before work', and you do this for a month, it becomes a habit and you don't need to think about it.
You create new neural pathways and connections in your mind.
Habits are shortcuts, so that you don't have to think.
Create a new pathway and it becomes subconscious.
Once the pathway is created, it's there and no longer requires a conscious decision.
You have taken it away from willpower.
Away from saying 'I know I should do… but I really want to… '

You often see people with addiction problems replacing old habits with new ones when they try to abstain from their addiction.
If you create a plan it will naturally become a habit over time.
It takes about four weeks to create a habit.
Before long it will become an everyday, normal part of your life that doesn't require thought.

Focus on eliminating the need for willpower.
Willpower is necessary to actually create a plan, but shouldn't be part of the plan.
When you rely on willpower you have not changed your lifestyle or subconscious thought pattern.

It is something you're going out of your way to do and you must rely on being highly motivated to sustain it.

Unfortunately, you will not be highly motivated about any one thing forever more.

You need a better solution.

Such as ingraining a habit.

You eliminate the need for willpower by having a plan that becomes a habit and that soon starts to become your lifestyle.

So it is now no longer reliant on you being highly conscious and motivated.

Take note when you have to make a decision.

If you have to make a decision, you're putting yourself in a difficult position.

Where you need to rely on willpower to ensure you go for the 'right' option.

Ideally you don't want to have to make any decisions at all when it comes to your health and fitness routines.

They should be just that – routine.

If you rely on willpower it's very easy to end up going round in circles and people often get trapped in an obsessive healthy versus binging cycle.

Try and create habits instead so you escape the negative cycle and good choices become as regular and familiar to you as brushing your teeth.

Failure = bad

On a psychological level, it's bad when you fail.

It reinforces negative thoughts about not being able to achieve your goals and being a failure.

When something goes wrong and your willpower fails, it can be damaging in the long term.

Remember: Failure usually simply means you don't have a good plan in place.

Take that as a lesson instead of a failure, then adjust your plan and continue as normal.

This will be psychologically much healthier for you than beating yourself up every time you 'fail'.

Treat yourself how you would treat somebody else.

Accumulate Little Wins

If you've never exercised before, trying to train five times a week is going to be too much for you. Aim to go at least once a week, every week, without fail.
You will start to build your confidence.
Once you've mastered it, increase it to twice a week.
There is no need to be in some great rush.
Of course, start where you are at and don't regress, but accumulate your small wins.
Start with something you know you can do.
Then do it.
Do it well.

Don't forget to celebrate these small wins.
These are your process goals.
Your outcome goal is the final piece of the puzzle, and your process goals are simply the achievement of following the plan.
Deciding and managing to go to the gym twice in one week is a process.
If you go twice a week consistently, then you should celebrate this.
Feel proud of your achievements.
Break your big, distant goal down into smaller weekly or even daily targets.
They're easy to hit and ensure you are always moving in the right direction.

If someone's diet is abysmal, trying to be perfect all the time is going to be difficult.
Just aim to get breakfast right every single day until the habit becomes normality.
Then work on lunch and then, gradually, after a few weeks, three quarters of your meals will be healthy.
You need the mindset that there is no such thing as failure.
That way, when something goes wrong you learn from it, but it doesn't mean you've failed.
It's a lesson.
It does not mean you are a failure, it just means you haven't achieved your goals yet.
Embrace it as a lesson, learn from it so you do not repeat your mistakes.
We cannot emphasise this enough.

Be Consistent, Always

Why are habits so fundamental that they take a whole chapter?
Because what you do consistently is what you become.
Managing habits is a means to your desired end.
More than that, it is absolutely essential to long term success.
When you have identified a change you wish to make, stick with it consistently for a sustained period of time and you will start to see the outcomes you are going for.
You need to practise consistency.
Initially it will often be difficult.
You have a lot of old habits and beliefs working against you.
The more you work at it, practise and persevere, the easier it becomes.
Anybody who tells you that it is easy is lying.
That doesn't mean it is hard forever, though.
Change is hard.
After change is made, it is your new normal.
Then it is easy.
Maintenance is easy.
You just need to fight to get there.

Do This: Download our compliance tracker (Page 180)

- Use it in conjunction with the weekly planner to track your progress.

- Are you doing what you have said you were going to do? Fill in the tracker and you will know.

- Compare the compliance to your outcome measurements to see how what you are doing is affecting the outcome.

- Modify one process goal at a time and track it using the compliance tracker.

CHECKLIST

Have you:
- ✓ **Set your process goals**
- ✓ **Completed your weekly log**
- ✓ **Completed the compliance tracker**

Summary

So there you have it.

The Five Pillars laid out and explained, along with a host of resources to facilitate you in accomplishing your goals over the next 30 days, and permanently.

Now all that is left is to do it.

If you have read this far, you have all of the information that you will need to be fit and healthy in just 30 minutes a day.

Remember that it is not an all or nothing deal.

Just do what you can and build from there.

It is just 30 minutes for 30 days…

If you have not started on the exercises included throughout the book yet, we urge you to begin now, whilst it is fresh in your mind.

Procrastinating never helped anybody achieve anything.

Below is a full checklist of all the exercises for you to go through.

Make sure that you have done them all now.

FULL CHECKLIST:

- ✓ Written your life story
- ✓ Completed the bridge model
- ✓ Re-written your long term goals
- ✓ Defined what measurements to use in tracking progress and taken measurement
- ✓ Filled in and signed the commitment sheet
- ✓ Blogged about your journey

- ✓ Understood the 'Eat this, not that' document
- ✓ Used the recipes e-book
- ✓ Planned your meals for the week
- ✓ Created weekly shopping lists
- ✓ Organised food deliveries

- ✓ Improved your sleep hygiene
- ✓ Booked restorative session
- ✓ Altered your products to natural alternatives
- ✓ Made time to relax and play

- ✓ Worked daily on mobility
- ✓ Structured your training calendar
- ✓ Completed interval cardio workouts
- ✓ Completed strength training workouts

- ✓ Written process goals
- ✓ Completed the weekly log
- ✓ Completed compliance tracker and used it to set new process goals

The Next Steps

Complete the 30 Day Plan as set out below. See the resources that follow for instructions on exactly what to do.

30 Day Plan

Day 1. Bridge model
Day 2. Training 1
Day 3. Life story
Day 4. Food guidelines – have healthy food
Day 5.Training 2
Day6. Measurements and I will… goals and process goals
Day 7. Food preparation
Day 8. Shopping
Day 9. Training 3
Day 10. Commitment sheet
Day 11. Training 4
Day 12. Restorative exercise
Day 13. Plan food, shopping
Day 14. Prepare food
Day 15. Training 5
Day 16. Improve sleep hygiene
Day 17. Weekly log
Day 18. Training 6
Day 19. Restorative exercise
Day 20. Contemplate your progress – 20 things you have achieved
Day 21. Prepare food
Day 22. Training 7
Day 23. Improve products
Day 24. Weekly log
Day 25. Training 8
Day 26. Restorative exercise
Day 27. Try a new exercise
Day 28. Prepare food
Day 29. Training 9
Day 30. Compliance tracker

Resources

Bridge model

Bridge Model

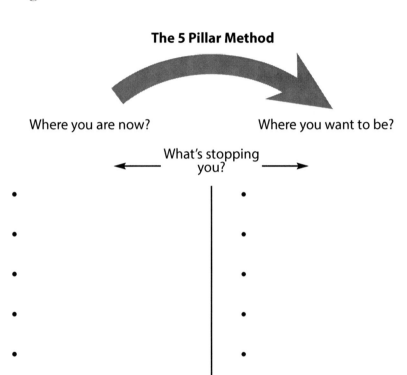

The 5 Pillar Method

Where you are now?   Where you want to be?

What's stopping you?

-
-
-
-
-
-

-
-
-
-
-

-
-
-
-

Training 1

See www.aretefitness.co.uk/exercises *for exercise demonstrations*

Order	Exercise	Sets	Reps	Rest
1	Hip Lifts	3	12	45 Seconds
2	Face Pulls	3	12	45 Seconds
3	Body Weight Squat	3	12	45 Seconds
4	Standing Dumbbell Press	3	12	45 Seconds
5	Dumbbell Split Squats	3	12	45 Seconds
6	Dumbbell Incline Chest Press	3	12	45 Seconds
7	Lat Pull Down	3	12	45 Seconds
8	Plank	3	12	45 Seconds

Your Life Story

This is a thought experiment to explore your deep values and subconscious desires. It will help you to understand what you want from life, both in health and fitness, and generally.

You are 40/60 years old. Write about your life. What are you known for? What do you do every day? Where do you live? How do you live? What have you achieved in your life? What are you working towards now? What is your proudest moment? Biggest regret? Talk about your home, family, hobbies, talk about work, talk about your passions.

Just start writing, and do not stop until you run out of things to say. You will answer lots of other questions too that are not mentioned here. When you shut your logical mind off and stop worrying about how any of this was possible, you will release a lot of things in your head you probably weren't conscious of.

The aim is to hit flow, do not read back or stop to consider what you are writing, just keep the pen moving until you have finished. Make sure you are writing the old fashioned way with pen and paper; this is important. It might not even all make sense when you have finished and read back, but that is fine.

Do not consider it before you start writing. Just start writing now.

There is no correct way to do this, just begin writing and see what comes out. The act of writing is the key.

DAY 4

Food guidelines - have healthy food

The aim of any healthy eating plan should be to create a diet that is enjoyable, simple, sustainable and fun!

The underlying principle of everything we recommend regarding diet is to eat real food. Food that your grandmother would recognise, food that is natural, that people have eaten since the dawn of time. Food that is nutrient-dense, tasty, health-promoting and energising.

We've tried to keep this guide short in the hope of not boring you, so we have skimmed over the 'why' quickly and concentrated on what you should be doing and how to do it.

We use a set of guidelines that you should aim to follow…

If, for whatever reason, things do go pear-shaped it is vital that first of all you do not let it get you down, and secondly that you get back on track at the next available opportunity.

Long term, sustainable results are achieved by increasing compliance on a realistic, sustainable program, not by using some crazy crash diet for a week and being back where you started a week later.

Real Food Guidelines

- Eat Protein At Breakfast – stabilise blood sugar and give sustained energy. *What is protein?* Any meat, fish, eggs or dairy. *What can I eat?* Eggs and smoked salmon, bacon and avocado, organic natural/Greek yoghurt and fruit/nuts, cheese, ham and tomatoes, omelettes.

- Avoid industrial seed oils in favour of natural oils – *What are industrial seed oils?* Soybean, sunflower, safflower, rapeseed, margarines, vegetable oils. Swap vegetable oils, sunflower oil and margarines for natural alternatives such as butter, olive oil, coconut oil, goose/duck fat.

- Avoid soy – once touted as a health food, it is now clear that it is anything but. Properly treated soy (tempeh and miso) is not such a big deal, however soybean oil, soy milk, tofu should be avoided. *What should I eat instead?* Real meat, dairy and fish.

- Eat natural food instead of processed food – *What should I eat?* Most meals should be a protein (meat, fish, eggs, cheese/yoghurt) with vegetables/salad, whilst snacks should be thought of as a normal meal, just smaller, such as nuts, fruit. **Real food**.

- Avoid sugar – *Where is sugar?* Everywhere in processed food, this one is mostly taken care of in the previous and following point.

- Avoid liquid calories – *Where are liquid calories?* Fizzy drinks, fruit juices, smoothies, milk, fancy coffees, alcohol. *What should I drink?* Water (plenty of), coffee, tea. If water is bland, squeeze the juice of a lemon or lime in it. Avoid caffeine late in the day.

- Anything labelled diet/low fat/lite/no fat is a scam. It is not healthy and will not help in weight loss or be healthy for you.

- Fat is not the enemy – Many fats are indeed necessary for good health and it is simply untrue that eating fat makes you fat. Does eating tuna make you a fish? *What are good sources of fat?* Butter, coconut oil, red meats, oily fish are all excellent sources of fat.

- Make better alcohol choices – *Didn't you already say avoid alcohol as liquid calories?* Yes, but nobody will listen! That's fine, however you can still make better choices, wine or clear spirits with minimal mixers (soda, tonic) will be much better than beers, cocktails, alcopops or anything with coke/orange juice.

Eat This, Not That

	Foods to include	Foods to exclude
Fruits	All fresh whole fruits	Dried fruit, fruit juice, smoothies
Vegetables	All fresh raw, steamed, boiled, sautéed, or roasted	
Starch	Sweet potato, all root veg (squash , pumpkin, swede etc.), potato, rice	Wheat, corn, barley, spelt, kamut, rye, oats, all gluten-containing products, quinoa
Legumes	Kidney, butter, & black beans etc., chickpeas, lentils, tempeh, miso	Soybeans, tofu, soy milk, baked beans, soy 'fake' meat
Nuts and seeds	All raw nuts	Roasted or salted nuts, seeds
Meat and fish	Fish, turkey, lamb, wild game, beef, chicken, pork	hotdogs, canned meat, sausages, meat substitutes made from soy
Dairy products and milk substitutes	cheese, thick cream (double, clotted), butter, yoghurt	Milk, ice cream, non-dairy creamers, low fat anything, soy milk, almond milk
Fats	Extra virgin olive oil, coconut oil, butter, goose/duck fat, olives, avocado, ghee	Margarine, processed and hydrogenated oils, mayonnaise, spreads
Beverages	Drink plenty of fresh water, herbal teas (e.g. rooibos, peppermint, etc.). Coffee – before 1400, Alcohol (wine, g&t, vodka+soda only)	Other alcohol, sodas, fizzy drinks (including diet drinks), fruit juice, smoothies, veg juices
Spices and condiments	Sea salt, fresh pepper, fresh herbs and spices (i.e. garlic, cumin, dill, ginger, oregano, parsley, rosemary, thyme, turmeric)	ketchup, soy sauce, barbecue sauce, other sauces
Sweeteners	Honey	White or brown sugar, maple syrup, corn syrup, high fructose corn syrup, desserts

Training 2

Weight Training Workout 2

Order	Exercise	Sets	Reps	Rest
1	Hip Lifts	3	12	45 Seconds
2	Face Pulls	3	12	45 Seconds
3	Body Weight Squat	3	12	45 Seconds
4	Standing Dumbbell Press	3	12	45 Seconds
5	Dumbbell Split Squats	3	12	45 Seconds
6	Dumbbell Incline Chest Press	3	12	45 Seconds
7	Lat Pull Down	3	12	45 Seconds
8	Plank	3	12	45 Seconds

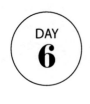

DAY 6

Measurements and I will... goals and process goals

Measurements

- What do you wish to change?

- How do you determine whether you are making changes in the right direction?

Answering these two questions will indicate what is it you should measure.

Keeping tabs on your progress is important for motivation and to know that what you are doing is working.

So, define what you can measure to keep track of your goals. Some ideas are below but you can use your own.

Strength   How many press ups you can do

Running   Your 5k time

Weight   Your dress size and girth measurement around waist, hips and thighs, body fat percentage

Energy   A scale of 1-10 how energised you feel: upon waking, mid-morning, after lunch, late afternoon

Health   Body fat percentage, energy, strengthYour

Outcome Goals

I Will...

Define your goals and put a date on them.

Examples:

I will... lose a dress size in six weeks

I will... be able to do 10 press ups in two months

I will... be able to do a pull up in six months

I will... set a new 5k personal best in four weeks

Process Goals

What do you need to do in order to achieve the goals stated above? There will probably be a number of process goals for each outcome goal. You should be able to set a process goal for every variable that will affect the outcome.

Examples:

I will… eat whole food from the guidelines at least 85% of the time for the next six weeks

I will… work on press ups three times a week until I can do 10

I will… work on my upper body strength three times a week, until I can do a pull up

I will… follow a 5k preparation running program

Food preparation

Food Preparation

On the food preparation days, you should spend time preparing healthy meals for the coming week. This could be chopping vegetables and marinating meat that will be used over the next couple of days; it could be cooking a large batch of something that can be reheated for lunch or preparing a huge salad that you can take for lunch for several days.

Examples:

- Chop vegetables and salad and keep in Tupperware so they are handy when you come home in the evening

- Marinate meats/fish to flavour, ready to cook.

- Batch cook a large meal such as chilli con carne, shepherd's pie, roast dinner that can be reheated/eaten cold in the following days

- Make a large salad that you can take for lunch the next three days

- Prepare breakfasts for the coming days to ensure you start the day off with a good meal

- Throw out processed foods that you no longer wish to eat and stock up on handy snacks such as nuts

Shopping

Shopping

If possible, go somewhere new (and healthy) such as the butchers, greengrocers, farmers market or fishmonger. Speak to them about how to cook new things, recipe ideas and combinations. The aim is to broaden the possibilities of things you can prepare.

If not possible, spend half an hour in the supermarket with a list of foods you are going to buy. Learn where the things are that you will be buying regularly and which aisles are full of stuff you should avoid. Fresh food is usually around the edges of a store with processed food in the aisles in the centre. Avoid going to the shops when hungry to minimise impulse purchases.

Alternatively, organise food delivery online and buy healthy foods for the week. Supermarkets offer this service and so do a number of butchers and grocers online. This is a great way to get high quality food if you do not have access to a good butcher or farmers market in your area – or do not have the time to go.

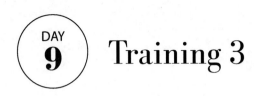

DAY 9 — Training 3

Cardio

The cardio program is a progressive plan which for Sessions 1 and 2 starts you off at a steady pace. The aim of these sessions is to introduce you back to cardio training and help you build fitness up for the interval plans in the following sessions.

In Session 1 you need to just go out there and start moving. The aim is to be training for a total of 20 minutes. Be it the treadmill, a swim, on a bike, or running in the park, get yourself working up a sweat. Session 2: do the same, but for 30 minutes. Depending on your base fitness levels you may be able to do these times without resting, , however, if you need to break, go slow, or walk during the session, do.

Time	Intensity
20	4/10

DAY 10 — Commitment Sheet

Commitment Sheet

Take your 'I will…' statements.
Underneath, sign and date them.
Have somebody else also sign and date them.
Somebody who you want to be accountable to – you should value their opinion and not want to let them down. By showing them your statements, you are becoming accountable to them on a subconscious level. You will not want to go against your word. Social accountability can be a strong influence on your actions, so do not underestimate the power of this exercise.

I will….
I will….
I will….
I will….

Sign   Date

Weight Training Workout 3

Order	Exercise	Sets	Reps	Rest
A1	Hip Lifts	3	12	None
A2	Face Pulls	3	12	45 Seconds
B1	Body Weight Squat	3	12	None
B2	Standing Dumbbell Press	3	12	45 Seconds
C1	Dumbbell Split Squats	3	12	None
C2	Dumbbell Incline Chest Press	3	12	45 Seconds
D1	Step Ups	3	12	None
D2	Plank	3	Max Time	45 Seconds
E1	Lat Pull Down	3	12	None
E2	Side Planks	3	Max Time	45 Seconds

DAY 12 · Restorative exercise

Restorative Exercise

Restorative exercise can take a number of forms including yoga, Pilates, tai chi, mindfulness and more.

You may well not have ever done any of these activities, so we encourage you to try something new.

You can take a class, or get a DVD to do at home.

A good suggestion is to get a friend and try out a new class together.

Plan food, shopping

Food Planning

It is important to not get bored of the same staple meals when you embark upon a healthier eating regime. It is very easy to rely on a couple of standard meals and get yourself in to a rut, which will inevitably be broken with a junk food binge.

Coming up are some examples of meals you could try for breakfast, lunch and dinner, as well as some healthy snacks and desserts. We highly encourage you to try new things out, discover new flavours and cuisines to keep it interesting and varied.

Breakfast Menu

Grab and Dash – preparation time under 1 minute

- Pack of cold meat, handful of nuts

- Leftover roast meat, Handful of berries

- Organic natural yoghurt, nuts/fruit

- Hardboiled eggs (prep ahead of time), smoked salmon/fruit/nuts

- Protein shake, nuts/fruit

- Cold fish (salmon, mackerel, sardines, tuna, etc.)

Hearty Meal – preparation time 2-10 minutes

- Bacon and eggs

- Scrambled eggs and tomatoes

- Parma ham and melon

- Bacon and avocado

- Reheat leftovers

- Cheese, ham and tomato

- Cheese, berries

- Nut butter/cream cheese/pate on celery/carrots

Gourmet Breakfast – preparation time 10+ minutes

- Full English (bacon, eggs, mushrooms, tomatoes)

- Omelettes

- Homemade burgers/patties, salad/avocado/egg

Lunch Menu

- Thai chicken, chorizo and feta with mixed leaves

- Tuna Niçoise salad

- Cooked prawns, smoked salmon or salmon fillets with mixed leaves, tomatoes, and avocado. Olive oil as a dressing

- Sliced meat from last night's dinner: roast beef, ham, any continental ham, chicken or turkey with leftover or raw veggies such as pepper, carrot, tomato

- Feta cheese Greek salad

- Tricolore salad – Mozzarella, avocado and tomato. Serve with fresh basil and an olive oil and balsamic vinegar dressing.

- Cottage cheese with beetroot, mixed leaves, pine nuts and olive oil

- Homemade beef stew (diced beef, stock, salt, pepper, onion, garlic, assorted root vegetables)

- Shepherds/cottage pie

- Fish pie (mashed squash topping)

- Jerk or spiced chicken, sweet potatoes and vegetables

- Homemade kebab skewers: chicken, beef or prawns with mixed veg – onions, peppers, mushrooms, tomato, courgette

Dinner Menu

Quick and Easy – preparation time 10 minutes or less

- Stir fry (pre-packed stir fry veg + diced meat/prawns, herbs/spices)

- Bell pepper stuffed with tuna + melted cheese

- Steak fried with onion & mushroom with green leaves

- Pre-prepared homemade burgers/patties with avocado slices and salad

- Gammon steak with egg/pineapple & salad

- Leftovers!

- Homemade microwave meals

Hearty and Nutritious – preparation time under 20 minutes

- Foil-baked salmon with ginger, spinach and pine nuts, beetroots

- Red/Green Thai curry (diced meat/fish, coconut milk/cream, assorted veggies such as peppers, broccoli, squash, onion, mushroom, curry paste, chilli, garlic, lemon/lime juice)

- Grilled fish with a selection of veggies

- Bone in chicken breast, baked with tomato, basil pesto, onions, garlic, with leek mash (leek, garlic, butter, mashed potato)

- Rack of lamb with green veggies

- Mexican 'fajita' mix (flash fry strips of meat, onions, peppers, tomatoes, spices) served over salad

- Organic/gluten free sausages (go to the butchers), mashed potato, butter, caramelised onions (fry in butter)

Here's One I Made Earlier – cook in bulk and eat cold/reheat for lunch or quick convenient evening meals

- Sunday roast (any joint with whatever veggies) – buy at least double what you need and have the rest for leftovers next breakfast/lunch/evening

- Chilli con carne (mince, tinned tomatoes, onion, mushroom, peppers, kidney beans, herbs/spices) – easy to freeze and reheat

- Homemade burgers/patties (mince, finely diced onion, garlic, chilli/herbs, 1 egg to bind) – pull out and grill, serve with avocado and salad

- Casserole (meat on the bone, root veggies, stock) – slow cook, freeze, then reheat for a quick, easy meal

- Chicken and onion soup (bake and shred chicken breast, fry onions until soft, throw in stock, seasoning and cook) – quick and easy to reheat

- Fish pie (fry fish pie mix, onions, mushrooms, garlic. Boil and mash butternut squash. Add mushroom soup to fish, top with mashed squash and bake) – really tasty reheated

- Stock (bones, for example remnants of a whole roast chicken, water, onion, carrot, salt, pepper) – slow cook and use as a base for casseroles/soups. It will freeze

Snacks Menu

Snacks: A snack should be approached the same way as any other meal, following the same guidelines and eating real, whole foods.

- Pate and raw vegetables (celery, carrot, etc.)

- Cheese and olives

- Boiled egg

- Sliced meat

- Berries/apples

- Dried/cured beef (biltong)

- Raw carrots, peppers, tomatoes etc.

- Natural yoghurt with berries

Dessert Menu

Ready in two seconds

- ¾ small chunks of Green & Blacks organic 85% chocolate

- Organic berries with organic thick cream (double or clotted)

- Cheese assortment with grapes, sliced apples, or carrot sticks

- Yoghurt with either berries, nuts or dark chocolate (as above)

Time to cook

- **Chocolate Brownies**

    1 cup xylitol (sugar substitute)

    6 organic eggs

    100 grams plus 50 grams of Green and Blacks 85% chocolate

    ½ teaspoon salt

    ½ teaspoon vanilla1/3 cup butter (organic), melted

    ½ cup sifted TIANA Organic Coconut Flour

    1 cup nuts, chopped (optional)

In a saucepan at low heat, blend together butter and 100 grams of chocolate. Remove from heat and let cool. In a bowl, mix together eggs, xylitol, salt and vanilla. Stir in cocoa mixture. Whisk coconut flour into batter until there are no lumps. Fold in nuts and crumble in other 50 grams of chocolate. Pour batter into a greased 11x7x2 or 8x8x2 inch pan. Bake at 175C (350F) for 30-35 minutes.

- **Pumpkin Muffins**

    1 ½ cups almond flour

    1 teaspoon baking powder

    1 teaspoon baking soda

    1 ½ teaspoons pumpkin pie spice, plus more for sprinkling on tops of muffins

    ⅛ teaspoon salt

    3 eggs

3 tablespoons honey

¾ cup canned pumpkin

1 small ripe banana, mashed

1 teaspoon vanilla extract

⅓ cup chopped pecans (plus more to sprinkle on top)

Preheat oven to 350F. Line muffin pan with paper liners or use coconut oil to grease pan.

In a large bowl, whisk together almond flour, baking powder, baking soda, pumpkin pie spice, and salt. Set aside.

In a small bowl, whisk together eggs, pumpkin, banana, and vanilla extract. Add wet ingredients to dry ingredients and mix to combine. Stir in pecans until well incorporated.

Scoop batter into prepared muffin pan cups filling ¾ full. Sprinkle the tops of the muffins with pecans and pumpkin pie spice.

Bake muffins for 20 to 25 minutes or until golden.

- **Grilled Bananas with Cinnamon**

  2 bananas, quarter, leave peel on

  Cinnamon

  Coconut oil

Brush the open side of the banana with coconut oil if desired then sprinkle on cinnamon to taste. Grill open side down (peel up) for 2-4 minutes, flip and grill peel down for another 2-4 minutes or until the peel starts to separate from the fruit. Remove from the grill and serve. It's fun to eat it out of the peel.

Prepare food

Food Preparation

On the food preparation days, you should spend time preparing healthy meals for the coming week. This could be chopping vegetables and marinating meat that will be used over the next couple of days; it could be cooking a large batch of something that can be reheated for lunch or preparing a huge salad that you can take for lunch for several days.

Examples:
- Chop vegetables and salad and keep in Tupperware so they are handy when you come home in the evening

- Marinate meats/fish to flavour, ready to cook.

- Batch cook a large meal such as chilli con carne, shepherd's pie, roast dinner that can be reheated/eaten cold in the following days

- Make a large salad that you can take for lunch the next three days

- Prepare breakfasts for the coming days to ensure you start the day off with a good meal

- Throw out processed foods that you no longer wish to eat and stock up on handy snacks such as nuts

Training 5

Weight Training Workout 4

Order	Exercise	Sets	Reps	Rest
A1	Hip Lifts	3	12	None
A2	Face Pulls	3	12	45 Seconds
B1	Body Weight Squat	3	12	None
B2	Standing Dumbbell Press	3	12	45 Seconds
C1	Dumbbell Split Squats	3	12	None
C2	Dumbbell Incline Chest Press	3	12	45 Seconds
D1	Step Ups	3	12	None
D2	Plank	3	Max Time	45 Seconds
E1	Lat Pull Down	3	12	None
E2	Side Planks	3	Max Time	45 Seconds

Improve sleep hygiene

Get Better Sleep

Sleep is consistently the most overlooked component of a healthy lifestyle. People know all about diet and exercise and they focus on these two components whilst overlooking or choosing to ignore other important pieces to the jigsaw of good health such as sleep and stress. When you sleep well, you recover from training quicker, maintain good insulin sensitivity, lower stress, normalise hormonal rhythms, have higher energy levels, a stronger immune system and general overall good health. To get the best possible night's sleep here are a few tips you can implement:

- Be consistent – whenever possible try to sleep and to wake at approximately the same times daily. Late nights should be an exception to the rule, not reason to consistently break them. Consistency leads to better hormonal health.

- Make your room pitch black – like… pitch black. Get some blackout blinds and turn electronics off. It makes a big difference to quality of sleep; the body cannot produce melatonin (sleep hormone) properly in the presence of artificial light.

- Relax before you go to bed – I'm sure you know you can't jump straight from working to sleeping, your mind is going at a million miles an hour. The same is true for other things such as watching TV or being on the computer. Before bed try having a bath or shower, reading, gentle music, stretching or spending time with your partner to wind down and enter a state of relaxation before you try and settle down.

- As best you can, follow a natural light cycle – This means try to get sunlight during the day (artificial office light doesn't cut it), take your lunch outside and during the evening have dimmed lights or gentle lamps on instead of full power overhead lights blaring at you. Your body reacts to light and dark hormonally; this is the reason that when it is sunny everybody automatically feels happier about life.

- Only get into bed when you are ready to sleep. Don't lie in bed watching TV, working on the laptop or chatting on your phone. You want the bed to be associated subconsciously with sleeping. You have a sofa for these other activities.

- Think happy thoughts before bed. Going to bed unhappy, nervous, agitated or angry will inhibit your ability to fall into restful sleep. Do something you enjoy, listen to uplifting music, or sit and think about the good things that have happened today before going to bed. It helps you relax and drift into a comfortable sleep.

Weekly log

Weekly Log

Record a few key areas which are relevant to your goals. This should be based on your process goals.
Some suggestions are: food, sleep, exercise, relaxation time.
Below are a couple of examples of how to do it.

Food Diary

The aim of a food diary is to measure exactly what you are eating and drinking over the course of a week. You will become much more aware of your own eating habits and you will see patterns emerge.
Be specific, write down exactly what you ate, what sauces/condiments/herbs/spices, what it is cooked in, what you drink, whether you bought or prepared yourself and whether you were at home/the office/restaurant.
Look over the diary at the end of each day and begin to correlate how you feel throughout the day with the foods you have eaten.

Monday

Meal	Location	Bought/ prepared	Food
Breakfast			
Lunch			
Dinner			
Snacks			
Drinks			

Sleep Diary

Record what time you get into bed, how much sleep you get, quality of sleep, how many times you woke in the night, how much energy you have upon waking.

Day	Bed time	Hours of sleep	Energy upon waking (1-10)	Times Woken	Quality of Sleep (1-10)
Monday					
Tuesday					
Wednesday					
Thursday					
Friday					
Saturday					
Sunday					

Exercise Diary

Record how many times per week and what type of training you complete. Build this into a habit of sustainable progression.

Day	Workout time	Workout type
Monday		
Tuesday		
Wednesday		
Thursday		
Friday		
Saturday		
Sunday		

Relaxation Diary

Record how much time you spend relaxing, winding down or doing something fun, and what this activity is. Examples include mindfulness, massage, walking, playing with kids/pet.

Day	Relaxation time	Activity	Happiness (1-10)
Monday			
Tuesday			
Wednesday			
Thursday			
Friday			
Saturday			
Sunday			

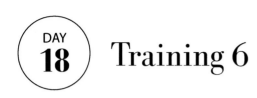

Training 6

Cardio Workout 2

Time	Intensity
30 mins	4/10

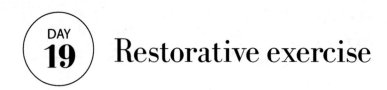

DAY 19 Restorative exercise

Restorative Exercise

Restorative exercise can take a number of forms including yoga, Pilates, tai chi, mindfulness and more.

You may well not have ever done any of these activities, so we encourage you to try something new.

You can take a class, or get a DVD to do at home.

A good suggestion is to get a friend and try out a new class together.

Contemplate your progress - 20 things you have achieved

20 Things I Have Achieved

Spend a little while contemplating some of the changes you have made in your life to this point, physically, practically, in your mindset, your beliefs. Write down a list of 20 things that you have achieved. Large or small, they are all significant.

This is a positively reinforcing exercise. It shows you how far you have come and keeps you motivated to continue progressing. You should celebrate small wins. It is the accumulation of small wins that leads to big results.

1.

2.

3.

4.

5.

6.

7.

8.

9.

10.

11.

12.

13.

14.

15.

16.

17.

18.

19.

20.

DAY 21 Prepare food

Food Preparation

On the food preparation days, you should spend time preparing healthy meals for the coming week. This could be chopping vegetables and marinating meat that will be used over the next couple of days; it could be cooking a large batch of something that can be reheated for lunch or preparing a huge salad that you can take for lunch for several days.

Examples:
- Chop vegetables and salad and keep in Tupperware so they are handy when you come home in the evening

- Marinate meats/fish to flavour, ready to cook.

- Batch cook a large meal such as chilli con carne, shepherd's pie, roast dinner that can be reheated/eaten cold in the following days

- Make a large salad that you can take for lunch the next three days

- Prepare breakfasts for the coming days to ensure you start the day off with a good meal

- Throw out processed foods that you no longer wish to eat and stock up on handy snacks such as nuts

DAY 22 — Training 7

Weight Training Workout 5

Order	Exercise	Sets	Reps	Rest
A1	Weighted Hip Lifts	3	12	None
A2	Face Pulls	3	12	60 Seconds
B1	Goblet Squat	3	12	None
B2	Dumbbell Press	3	12	60 Seconds
C1	Dumbbell Split Squats	3	12	None
C2	Dumbbell Incline Chest Press	3	12	60 Seconds
D1	Step Ups with Balance	3	12	None
D2	Plank – Back & Forth	3	Max Time	60 Seconds
E1	Lat Pull Down	3	12	None
E2	Triceps Push Downs	3	12	60 Seconds

DAY 23 — Improve products

Improve products

Improve Products

Do you have the slim waist and toned shoulders for the perfect hourglass figure, but the hips and thighs that make your shape decidedly more pear?

The reason you are disproportionally storing your body fat around the lower half of your body is oestrogen dominance – that is an excess of the female sex hormone oestrogen in your body, and/or you are not effectively clearing it from your body.

So What Causes This?

- High levels of environmental oestrogens in the body – Oestrogen is a natural, essential hormone, for both men and women, although in differing amounts between the sexes. Your body should produce and should also eliminate it after use (see the next point). Problems arise when you are exposed to high levels of environmental oestrogenous substances and your body gets overwhelmed with too much oestrogen versus its counter hormones such as progesterone and testosterone. Environmental oestrogens are everywhere nowadays and are putting an undue burden on your body. Some of the places they're found include soya foods and oils, beauty products, cleaning products, food and drink packaging, plastics, low quality meat and dairy products, pesticides, birth control and hormone replacement therapies.

- These environmental oestrogenous substances are known as xenoestrogens or endocrine disruptors; they're not real hormones but are similar in structure and thus bind to the same receptor sites in the body, they're often much stronger than the natural hormones your body would produce, having a more pronounced effect than even an equal amount of natural hormone. Unfortunately, more and more are making their way into the environment and our bodies are just not adapted to cope with them.

- Poorly liver: the inability to detoxify – hormones work on a cyclical basis, as do most things in the body. When a hormone is produced, in the ovaries in the case of oestrogen, it spreads through the body, fulfils its function and should then be eliminated. One of over 500 functions fulfilled by the liver is to break down old hormones and environmental toxins to a form that can be safely carried out of the body in the urine or faeces. If your liver is unable to efficiently do its job, the toxins cannot be broken down and cannot just 'hang around' because they're toxic! So they are put somewhere safe until such time that your body can better cope with breaking them down. The safe place, unfortunately, is in your fat stores. Looking after your liver can produce almost unbelievably quick drops in body fat levels, especially around the hips and thighs.

What Can I Do About It?

- Do not eat soya! It is bad for you in many more ways than just its oestrogen mimicking. Soy was originally fed to cattle because it fattened them up quicker than traditional feed... it also made them sick and they could only use it for three months before the animals started dying. Focus, instead, on meats, fish and eggs to get the full complement of essential proteins.

- Aim to eat the best quality foods you can afford/find. As mentioned in the previous point, soya is a cheap, efficient way to fatten up animals quickly. Try to find grass fed/pasture-raised animals and wild-caught fish; it costs a little more, but is definitely worth the investment. If you are eating commercially raised animals, look for leaner cuts because toxins are stored in the fat. Look for organic fruits and veggies that grow above the ground to avoid the pesticides. It is not so important for underground veggies such as onions, potatoes etc.

- Do not heat plastic containers – xenoestrogens leach from plastic containers into your food/drinks when heated. Don't microwave Tupperware containers, eat ready meals (obviously), or leave water bottles in the sun. It is recommended you do not re-use the same bottles/containers for too long as the materials degrade over time.

- Use natural products – the skin is the body's biggest organ. When you consider how many products people commonly use, from moisturisers, soaps, make-up, creams, deodorants, hair spray, shampoo, etc. and you also consider what is *in* these things you have to wonder what you are putting your body through. Read the ingredients on the nearest beauty product and I bet you can't even pronounce most of them, let alone know what they are. These chemicals are all being absorbed through the skin and entering your circulation. Whilst we don't recommend not using soap and deodorant, we do recommend using natural products that contain minimal, herbal type ingredients that have been successfully used for thousands of years. Some would say you should not put anything on your skin you would not put in your mouth... we do not recommend eating your soap, but the principle applies as it ultimately all ends up in the same place: in your body.

- Be aware of the effects birth control pills can have – we're not here to be making any recommendations about that sort of thing, however, we would like to make you aware that, firstly, it is not natural to flood your system with hormones and, secondly, it *will* have an effect on your health, weight and body composition.

- Lower your toxic load – when the liver is not overloaded with work it will do its job much more efficiently. Alcohol is a big toxic load; lowering intake will benefit everybody. Caffeine can also be an issue. Both in moderation are manageable, but chronic high level consumption will be an issue. Transfats or hydrogenated oils such as those in margarines and most processed food are extremely toxic, so a focus on real food is essential. Every point mentioned previously is going to help lower the toxic load your body has to deal with.

- Support your liver – fibre helps move things out of the body, so a diet containing plenty of veggies is a good place to start. Drink plenty of water, at least 2 litres a day, and eat food high in nutrients, such as grass fed meat and dairy, wild caught fish and organic veg. Exercising regularly helps remove waste products by increasing peripheral blood flow and sweating. Aim for at least three times a week. Along the same lines, a sauna is a good detoxifying tool. Certain nutritional supplements such as milk thistle and calcium D- glucarate are beneficial in supporting liver function.

- Eat your broccoli – cruciferous veggies such as broccoli, cauliflower, brussel sprouts, cabbage and kale contain a compound called diindolylmethan or DIM that is similar in structure to oestrogen, but about 1000 times less potent. DIM bind onto oestrogen receptors by the same mechanism as the bad xenoestrogens,, displacing the endocrine inhibitors. DIM is also available in supplemental form.

- Every time you use chemical-filled products, you are piling toxins in to your system and these accumulate over time, creating cellulite and causing fat gain around the hips and thighs. Choose wisely.

Weekly log

Weekly Log

Record a few key areas which are relevant to your goals. This should be based on your process goals.
Some suggestions are: food, sleep, exercise, relaxation time.
Below are a couple of examples of how to do it.

Food Diary

The aim of a food diary is to measure exactly what you are eating and drinking over the course of a week. You will become much more aware of your own eating habits and you will see patterns emerge.
Be specific, write down exactly what you ate, what sauces/condiments/herbs/spices, what it is cooked in, what you drink, whether you bought or prepared yourself and whether you were at home/the office/restaurant.
Look over the diary at the end of each day and begin to correlate how you feel throughout the day with the foods you have eaten.

Monday

Meal	Location	Bought/ prepared	Food
Breakfast			
Lunch			
Dinner			
Snacks			
Drinks			

Sleep Diary

Record what time you get into bed, how much sleep you get, quality of sleep, how many times you woke in the night, how much energy you have upon waking.

Day	Bed time	Hours of sleep	Energy upon waking (1-10)	Times Woken	Quality of Sleep (1-10)
Monday					
Tuesday					
Wednesday					
Thursday					
Friday					
Saturday					
Sunday					

Exercise Diary

Record how many times per week and what type of training you complete. Build this into a habit of sustainable progression.

Day	Workout time	Workout type
Monday		
Tuesday		
Wednesday		
Thursday		
Friday		
Saturday		
Sunday		

Relaxation Diary

Record how much time you spend relaxing, winding down or doing something fun, and what this activity is. Examples include mindfulness, massage, walking, playing with kids/pet.

Day	Relaxation time	Activity	Happiness (1-10)
Monday			
Tuesday			
Wednesday			
Thursday			
Friday			
Saturday			
Sunday			

Weight Training Workout 6

Order	Exercise	Sets	Reps	Rest
A1	Weighted Hip Lifts	3	12	None
A2	Face Pulls	3	12	60 Seconds
B1	Goblet Squat	3	12	None
B2	Dumbbell Push Press	3	12	60 Seconds
C1	Dumbbell Split Squats	3	12	None
C2	Dumbbell Incline Chest Press	3	12	60 Seconds
D1	Step Ups with Balance	3	12	None
D2	Plank – Back & Forth	3	Max Time	60 Seconds
E1	Lat Pull Down	3	12	None
E2	Triceps Push Downs	3	12	60 Seconds

DAY 26 — Restorative exercise

Restorative Exercise

Restorative exercise can take a number of forms including yoga, Pilates, tai chi, mindfulness and more.

You may well not have ever done any of these activities, so we encourage you to try something new.

You can take a class, or get a DVD to do at home.

A good suggestion is to get a friend and try out a new class together.

Try a new exercise

Try a New Exercise

It is important to keep an interest in your fitness, and not see it as a chore or mundane and repetitive.

A great way to keep it interesting and exciting is to try something new. Grab a friend who is up for it and try a new sport, class or workout.

Try a Crossfit class, go rock climbing, play ultimate Frisbee, whatever takes your fancy. Try new things and find something that you enjoy and can get in to.

DAY 28 Prepare food

Food Preparation

On the food preparation days, you should spend time preparing healthy meals for the coming week. This could be chopping vegetables and marinating meat that will be used over the next couple of days; it could be cooking a large batch of something that can be reheated for lunch or preparing a huge salad that you can take for lunch for several days.

Examples:

- Chop vegetables and salad and keep in Tupperware so they are handy when you come home in the evening

- Marinate meats/fish to flavour, ready to cook.

- Batch cook a large meal such as chilli con carne, shepherd's pie, roast dinner that can be reheated/eaten cold in the following days

- Make a large salad that you can take for lunch the next three days

- Prepare breakfasts for the coming days to ensure you start the day off with a good meal

- Throw out processed foods that you no longer wish to eat and stock up on handy snacks such as nuts

Training 9

Cardio Workout 3

In the third workout and onwards, we move on to interval cardio training. Using a treadmill is best for this as it allows you to see the exact pace you are running at. The third cardio session is all about finding the quickest pace you can go for 40 seconds. So do four minutes warming up at a steady pace; then go as quick as you can for 40 seconds. If you managed to complete the 40 seconds at that pace without stopping or slowing greatly, on the next interval go quicker. If you couldn't complete the 40 seconds, go slower.

To try the new pace you must first get your energy back by going slow for four minutes. Then go for it again for 40 seconds. Again, if you complete it, after the next four minutes recovering at a slower pace, go up to a quicker speed for another 40 second burst, and so on. Do four quick sprints in all, this should be enough to find you max speed.

Week 3 – Session 2   **Test day to find your maximum speed for 40 seconds**

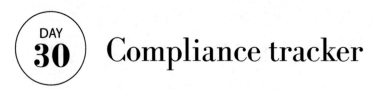

Compliance tracker

The compliance tracker is online and can be downloaded at
www.aretefitness.co.uk/compliance

Training Programs with exercise demonstrations – also available
online at www.aretefitness.co.uk/exercises

Training Plans

We recommend two to three weight-training sessions per week and up to two cardio sessions per week.

Weight Training

Weight Training Workout 1

Order	Exercise	Sets	Reps	Rest
1	Hip Lifts	3	12	45 Seconds
2	Face Pulls	3	12	45 Seconds
3	Body Weight Squat	3	12	45 Seconds
4	Standing Dumbbell Press	3	12	45 Seconds
5	Dumbbell Split Squats	3	12	45 Seconds
6	Dumbbell Incline Chest Press	3	12	45 Seconds
7	Lat Pull Down	3	12	45 Seconds
8	Plank	3	12	45 Seconds

Exercises
You will find photos of all the following exercises on www.aretefitness.co.uk/exercises

Hip Lifts

For this exercise you need a step or a bench.
Initiate the movement by squeezing the buttocks muscles and pushing through the heels to raise the hips up, until knees, hips and shoulders are all in alignment.
Slowly lower the hips back to the floor under control.

Face Pulls

Set the cables with a rope attachment in line with the top of your head. Stand tall with chest high and shoulders pulled back. Pull the rope towards the eyes, squeezing the shoulder blades together tightly and rotating the arms over. Pause at this point for a second.
Control the rope back to the start position. Make sure the posture is still tight and the shoulder blades are pulled back with each rep.

Squats

Stand with feet shoulder width apart and turned slightly out, and the chest high. Tighten the stomach muscles. This position should be maintained throughout the set.
Start the squat by pushing the knees out and sitting the hips down. Remember to keep the chest high. Squat as far down as possible, the aim should be to get all the way down so the hips are below the knees.
At the bottom, drive up by pushing your heels down and pull your hips through, squeezing your buttocks at the top.

Standing Dumbbell Press

Stand tall with shoulders pulled back and stomach muscles tight. The feet should be shoulder width apart. Hold the dumbbells by the shoulders. Press the weights over the head and together explosively. Lower under control back to the start position.

Dumbbell Split Squat

Stand with one foot in front of the other and shoulder width apart. Keep the chest high and abs tight.
Bend both knees until the back knee is just above the ground. Pause at the bottom for a second. Then drive up quickly, pushing through the front heel and returning to the start position.

Dumbbell Incline Chest Press

Set up a bench with an incline. Set feet slightly wider than shoulders to offer a steady base to press from. Start with the arms straight, separate the hands, slowly lower the dumbbells beside the shoulders.
At the bottom, take a slight pause, and then press the dumbbells back to the start point.

Lat Pull Down

Sit tall with the shoulders pulled back and chest high. Hold the bar with a slightly wider than shoulder width grip and pull the bar in towards the chest. Think about moving the elbows to the ribs.
Pause with the bar pulled tight at the bottom for a second before controlling the bar on the way up, back to the start.

Plank

Place the elbows on the floor underneath the shoulders and the legs out straight. When in the plank position, make sure the hips stay level by squeezing the stomach muscles and buttocks.
If you feel your hips drop, finish the set and then aim to increase the time in the next session. The aim is keeping a stable and controlled position.

Weight Training Workout 2

Order	Exercise	Sets	Reps	Rest
1	Hip Lifts	3	12	45 Seconds
2	Face Pulls	3	12	45 Seconds
3	Body Weight Squat	3	12	45 Seconds
4	Standing Dumbbell Press	3	12	45 Seconds
5	Dumbbell Split Squats	3	12	45 Seconds
6	Dumbbell Incline Chest Press	3	12	45 Seconds
7	Lat Pull Down	3	12	45 Seconds
8	Plank	3	12	45 Seconds

Exercises

Hip Lifts

For this exercise you need a step or a bench.
Initiate the movement by squeezing the buttocks muscles and pushing through the heels to raise the hips up, until knees, hips and shoulders are all in alignment.
Slowly lower the hips back to the floor under control.

Face Pulls

Set the cables with a rope attachment in line with the top of your head. Stand tall with chest high and shoulders pulled back. Pull the rope towards the eyes, squeezing the shoulder blades together tightly and rotating the arms over. Pause at this point for a second.

Control the rope back to the start position. Make sure the posture is still tight and the shoulder blades are pulled back with each rep.

Squats

Stand with feet shoulder width apart and turned slightly out, and the chest high. Tighten the stomach muscles. This position should be maintained throughout the set.
Start the squat by pushing the knees out and sitting the hips down. Remember to keep the chest high. Squat as far down as possible: the aim should be to get all the way down so the hips are below the knees.
At the bottom, drive up by pushing your heels down and pull your hips through, squeezing your buttocks at the top.

Standing Dumbbell Press

Stand tall with shoulders pulled back and stomach muscles tight. The feet should be shoulder width apart. Hold the dumbbells by the shoulders. Press the weights over the head and together explosively. Lower under control back to the start position.

Dumbbell Split Squat

Stand with one foot in front of the other and shoulder width apart. Keep the chest high and abs tight.
Bend both knees until the back knee is just above the ground. Pause at the bottom for a second. Then drive up quickly, pushing through the front heel and returning to the start position.

Dumbbell Incline Chest Press

Set up a bench with an incline. Set feet slightly wider than shoulders to offer a steady base to press from. Start with the arms straight, separate the hands, slowly lower the dumbbells beside the shoulders.
At the bottom, take a slight pause and then press the dumbbells back to the start point.

Lat Pull Down

Sit tall with the shoulders pulled back and chest high. Hold the bar with a slightly wider than shoulder width grip and pull the bar in towards the chest. Think about moving the elbows to the ribs.
Pause with the bar pulled tight at the bottom for a second before controlling the bar on the way up, back to the start.

Plank

Place the elbows on the floor underneath the shoulders and the legs out straight. When in the plank position, make sure the hips stay level by squeezing the stomach muscles and buttocks.
If you feel your hips drop, finish the set and then aim to increase the time in the next session. The aim is keeping a stable and controlled position.

Weight Training Workout 3

Order	Exercise	Sets	Reps	Rest
A1	Hip Lifts	3	12	None
A2	Face Pulls	3	12	45 Seconds
B1	Body Weight Squat	3	12	None
B2	Standing Dumbbell Press	3	12	45 Seconds
C1	Dumbbell Split Squats	3	12	None
C2	Dumbbell Incline Chest Press	3	12	45 Seconds
D1	Step Ups	3	12	None
D2	Plank	3	Max Time	45 Seconds
E1	Lat Pull Down	3	12	None
E2	Side Planks	3	Max Time	45 Seconds

New Exercises

Step Ups

Find a box or high step and begin with one foot on the box. This knee
should be bent beyond 90 degrees. From the start position, step up onto
the box by pushing through the heel of the top foot.
Stand tall on top, then step carefully back down to the start position.

Side Plank (option on knees)

You have an option here. Depending on training experience and fitness levels, either start the side plank on the feet or knees. Set the bottom elbow underneath the shoulders and the legs out straight. Raise the hips in line with the shoulders.

Again, this is about control and staying stable; to do so, keep the buttocks and abs tight. If the hips start to drop, stop and aim to increase the time next time.

Weight Training Workout 4

Order	Exercise	Sets	Reps	Rest
A1	Hip Lifts	3	12	None
A2	Face Pulls	3	12	45 Seconds
B1	Body Weight Squat	3	12	None
B2	Standing Dumbbell Press	3	12	45 Seconds
C1	Dumbbell Split Squats	3	12	None
C2	Dumbbell Incline Chest Press	3	12	45 Seconds
D1	Step Ups	3	12	None
D2	Plank	3	Max Time	45 Seconds
E1	Lat Pull Down	3	12	None
E2	Side Planks	3	Max Time	45 Seconds

In Workout 3 onwards we use supersets. Within the program of supersets we refer to reps and sets again, and introduce A1, A2 notation. A1 and A2 refer to the different exercise within a superset.

For example, superset a pair's hip lifts and face pulls. You do 12 reps of the hip lifts, or A1, followed straight away by 12 reps of the face pulls, or A2. A1 and A2 make one set of the superset. Rest for 45 seconds. Then repeat these three times to make three sets. Then move onto the next superset, B1 and B2.

New Exercises

Step Ups

Find a box or high step and begin with one foot on the box. This knee should be bent beyond 90 degrees. From the start position, step up onto the box by pushing through the heel of the top foot.
Stand tall on top, then step carefully back down to the start position.

Side Plank (option on knees)

You have an option here. Depending on training experience and fitness levels, either start the side plank on the feet or knees. Set the bottom elbow underneath the shoulders and the legs out straight. Raise the hips in line with the shoulders.
Again this is about control and staying stable, to do so keep the buttocks and abs tight. If the hips start to drop, stop and aim to increase the time next time.

Weight Training Workout 5

Order	Exercise	Sets	Reps	Rest
A1	Weighted Hip Lifts	3	12	None
A2	Face Pulls	3	12	60 Seconds
B1	Goblet Squat	3	12	None
B2	Dumbbell Press	3	12	60 Seconds
C1	Dumbbell Split Squats	3	12	None
C2	Dumbbell Incline Chest Press	3	12	60 Seconds
D1	Step Ups with Balance	3	12	None
D2	Plank – Back & Forth	3	Max Time	60 Seconds
E1	Lat Pull Down	3	12	None
E2	Triceps Push Downs	3	12	60 Seconds

New Exercises

Weighted Hip Lifts

Set yourself in a similar position as previously, but in this progression hold a weight securely on top of the hips. Again, lift the hips by squeezing the buttocks and driving through the heels.
As you drive the hips up make sure you hold the weight securely. Squeeze the buttocks at the top before lowering the hips back to the floor.

Goblet Squat

Stand with the feet shoulder width apart and turned slightly out. Grab the dumbbell in two hands by one end. Lift the chest by pulling the shoulders back and tighten the abs. This position should be held throughout the set. Start the squat by pushing the knees out and sitting the hips down. Squat as far down as possible. Your aim should be to get all the way down so the hips are below the knees. At the bottom, drive up by pushing the heels down and pull the hips through, squeezing the buttock muscles at the top.

Dumbbell Push Press

Stand tall with the feet shoulder width apart, shoulders pulled back and stomach tight. The first movement is down into a small squat, and then drive quickly up out of the squat using the momentum to help press the weights above the head.
Lower the weights back to the start position and go again.

Step Ups with Balance

This is a progression on the Step Ups earlier. Set yourself in a similar way. However, in this version the knee of the free foot comes up to the position shown below.
Hold this balance for one second or until you have complete control over your body. Then step carefully back down to the start position.

Plank with Forwards and Backwards Rock

Set yourself in a standard plank. In this progression, move the body back and forth by rocking on the toes. Keep the abs and buttocks tight and make sure the hips don't drop or stick up in the air.
Go as far in both directions as you can with good form and stop when you can no longer maintain good posture and control.

Triceps Push Down

Set the cable from the top with a rope attachment. Keep the elbows tucked in and make sure the shoulders stay pulled back. Push the handles down, straightening the elbows and squeezing the muscle at the back of the arm.
Control the handles back to the start position.

Weight Training Workout 6

Order	Exercise	Sets	Reps	Rest
A1	Weighted Hip Lifts	3	12	None
A2	Face Pulls	3	12	60 Seconds
B1	Goblet Squat	3	12	None
B2	Dumbbell Push Press	3	12	60 Seconds
C1	Dumbbell Split Squats	3	12	None
C2	Dumbbell Incline Chest Press	3	12	60 Seconds
D1	Step Ups with Balance	3	12	None
D2	Plank – Back & Forth	3	Max Time	60 Seconds
E1	Lat Pull Down	3	12	None
E2	Triceps Push Downs	3	12	60 Seconds

New Exercises

Weighted Hip Lifts

Set yourself in a similar position as previously, but in this progression hold a weight securely on top of the hips. Again, lift the hips by squeezing the buttocks and driving through the heels.
As you drive the hips up make sure you hold the weight securely. Squeeze the buttocks at the top before lowering the hips back to the floor.

Goblet Squat

Stand with the feet shoulder width apart and turned slightly out. Grab the dumbbell in two hands by one end. Lift the chest by pulling the shoulders back and tighten the abs. This position should be held throughout the set. Start the squat by pushing the knees out and sitting the hips down. Squat as far down as possible. Your aim should be to get all the way down so the hips are below the knees. At the bottom, drive up by pushing the heels down and pull the hips through, squeezing the buttock muscles at the top.

Dumbbell Push Press

Stand tall with the feet shoulder width apart, shoulders pulled back and stomach tight. The first movement is down into a small squat, and then drive quickly up out of the squat using the momentum to help press the weights above the head.
Lower the weights back to the start position and go again.

Step Ups with Balance

This is a progression on the Step Ups earlier. Set yourself in a similar way. However, in this version the knee of the free foot comes up to the position shown below.
Hold this balance for one second or until you have complete control over your body. Then step carefully back down to the start position.

Plank with Forwards and Backwards Rock

Set yourself in a standard plank. In this progression, move the body back and forth by rocking on the toes. Keep the abs and buttocks tight and make sure the hips don't drop or stick up in the air.
Go as far in both directions as you can with good form and stop when you can no longer maintain good posture and control.

Triceps Push Down

Set the cable from the top with a rope attachment. Keep the elbows tucked in and make sure the shoulders stay pulled back. Push the handles down, straightening the elbows and squeezing the muscle at the back of the arm.
Control the handles back to the start position.

The Authors

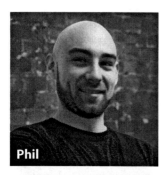

Phil

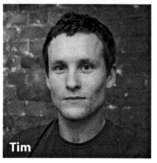

Tim

After taking very different paths to creating Arete fitness, Tim and Phil both share one major passion, their shared drive or 'why' in life. Tim came from a job working as a financial futures trader in The City of London, disliking the environment, finding the culture uncomfortable and ultimately not discovering the success he craved. He was never going to find his lives passion in such a place.

Phil grew up in the northern industrial town of Scunthorpe surrounded by little sense of possible achievement, drive or ambition. Phil was determined not to let this affect his life and his 'why'.

A 'why' is why you do what you do, why you get up in the morning, why you love it, your passion in life.

When they met they realised that they both shared the same 'why', that was to help as many people as possible to take control of their health; love exercise, eat positively and be strong, both physically and mentally.

From this passion Arete Fitness was born. Arete is charged with reinvigorating the outdated perception of female health and fitness, 30 minutes at a time.

Along the journey of writing this book they have become leaders in the health and fitness industry. Between them they have featured as experts in The Sunday Times, The Daily Mail, Women's Fitness, The Daily Express and more.

Both are passionate writers and blog their thoughts and ideas regularly on their personal websites www.TimDrummond.com and www.PhilHawksworth.com, as well as www.Aretefitness.co.uk.

Lightning Source UK Ltd.
Milton Keynes UK
UKOW05f0659180913

217402UK00001B/10/P